Potcakes

New Directions in the Human-Animal Bond

Alan M. Beck, series editor

Potcakes

Dog Ownership in New Providence, The Bahamas

William J. Fielding

Jane Mather

Maurice Isaacs

Purdue University Press
West Lafayette, Indiana

Library of Congress Cataloging-in-Publication Data

Fielding, William J., 1956–
  Potcakes : dog ownership in New Providence, the Bahamas / William J. Fielding, Jane
Mather, Maurice Isaacs.
     p. cm. -- (New discoveries in human-animal links)
  Includes bibliographical references and index.
  ISBN 1-55753-334-2
  1. Dogs--Bahamas--New Providence Island. 2. Dogs--Social aspects--Bahamas--New
Providence Island. 3. Dog owners--Bahamas--New Providence Island. 4. Human-animal
relationships--Bahamas--New Providence Island. I. Mather, Jane. II. Isaacs, Maurice.
III. Title. IV. Series.

  SF422.6.B24F54 2005
  636.7'009729'6--dc22

                                                                    2004021845

Dedicated to our tolerant "better halves,"
Solange, Robert, & Charlene
and WF's Rachel & Jonathan

Contents

Acknowledgments

This volume was only possible as a result of assistance of a great many people and groups, and we owe them all thanks.

The Department of Agriculture instigated and funded the perception study in New Providence, and so was the prime mover behind this publication. Consequently, we are delighted that the Minister of Agriculture, Fisheries and Local Government, the Honourable V. Alfred Gray M.P. has provided us with a foreword and given this book his support. We are also indebted to Carl Smith and Valerie Outten of the Department of Agriculture for their interest and encouragement in these studies.

John Hammerton was responsible for first getting WF to join the Animal Control Unit's Stray Dog Committee, chaired by M.I. It was this association that started WF investigating the dog population in New Providence, as well as providing the forum for the meeting of the authors. The work of the Stray Dog Committee also received valuable input from JM, Ton Vlugman (Pan American Health Organization) and Derrick Bailey (Department of Agriculture) in planning the resident perception study.

These studies have been made with the intention of putting issues associated with dogs on a systematic foundation. Our efforts have benefited immeasurably from much welcome advice from Alan Beck, of Purdue University and Andrew Rowan, of the Humane Society of the United States. Both have taken active interest in our work and provided technical, as well as moral support for our investigations. Their help in our studies cannot be underestimated. We also thank Alan for encouraging us to write this book.

We are grateful to the Department of Agriculture, the Princess Margaret Hospital, the Human Society of United States, the Bahamas Humane Society (in particular Suzette Hepburn-Lyn, Percy Grant and Stephen Turnquest), the Bahamas Kennel Club (in particular June Hall and Rita Hall), Brenda Franke of Animal House, Animals Require Kindness (Donna Kiriaze and Caroline Brogden) and veterinarians (in particular Patrick Balfe, Peter Bizzell, Gary Cash, Basil Sands and Dawn Wilson) for data which have provided useful insights into dog ownership. We are grateful to Baldwin Carey and Kayla Musgrove of the Department of Public Health for making possible the study on dog related disorders and human health. Livingston Hepburn (Department of Environmental Health Service) kindly arranged for data to be recorded on the numbers of dead dogs collected by Solid Waste Collection. We are also grateful to the staff at the Animal Control Unit for their help in many aspects of these studies. Sally Gamble and Vanessa Eneas assisted with the data collect of the resident perception study in New Providence. Chris and Molly Roberts (Abaco Animals Require Friends), Linda Giovino and Glenn Albury, and David Knowles (Department of Agriculture) assisted with the studies in Marsh Harbour, Abaco. The studies in Abaco were supported by the Humane Society International. Alan Davis, Animal Care & Regulation Division, Broward

County, Florida, assisted us on issues relating to dog disorders. John Gibb (Pan-American Health Organization) enabled us to gain access to World Health Organization reports on dogs.

We are grateful to many staff at The College of The Bahamas who have contributed to our investigations. In particular, Pandora Johnson (Research, Planning & Development) showed much interest in our work and Joan Vanderpool (Research Unit), who supported our efforts and engaged in lively discussion. Cristin Carole (School of Education) involved her students in pet studies, and with assistance of Joan Vanderpool and Denise Samuels (Research Unit) conducted focus groups with students on pet issues. Willamae Johnson and Berthmae Walker and the College Librarians encouraged students to participate in the studies, and Susan Plumridge (School of Social Sciences) asked her students about the meaning of "potcake", supervised a student project on animal cruelty, and assisted in the preliminary study on dogs as protectors. Her students also collected data on the study concerning tourists. Gloria Gomez (School of Education) provided access to a student project on roaming dogs. Florence Lawlor (School of English Studies) assisted us in compiling the description of New Providence, and other historical aspects, and Jessica Minnis, (School of Social Sciences) assisted with the interpretation of the social context of our results. Virginia Ballance (Hilda Bowen Library) found many useful articles and pictures and was constantly encouraging. Denise Samuels assisted in data collect and brought various aspects of the potcake in society to our attention. Janet Donnelly (School of English) provided leads on the origin of the word "potcake."

We also extend thanks to those who helped with our archival searches. These include the staff in the Special Collection at the library of The College of The Bahamas, the staff at the Department of Archives, in particular Gail Saunders and Lulamae Gray. In addition, Christopher Bates of "The Tribune" archives assisted in finding articles and photographs and Jim Lawlor who kindly drew our attention to many useful articles in the course of his own archival research.

Gail Saunders kindly read and commented upon an earlier draft of the chapter on dogs in New Providence and Andrea Beetz read the section on pet attachment. We are also grateful to Madeleine Malenczuk, who helped with proofreading an early draft. And, of course, we are grateful to the many hundreds of people who filled out questionnaires, allowed themselves to be interviewed and so provided the bulk of the data reported here.

We owe special thanks to the staff at Purdue University Press for their patience and tolerance during the preparation of the book. We are also very grateful to our families who supported us during our studies.

World Health Organization publications are used with the permission. The poem "The Potcake in Me" by Marion Bethel is copyrighted and reproduced with permission. Lyrics to "Who Will Love the Potcake?" sung by Lovey Forbes, were written by Joy DiAntonio, and those to "Mix-up Dog" by Eddie Minnis. Both these songs are copyrighted and reproduced with permission. "The Cry of the Potcake" is copyrighted and was written and sung by Phil Stubbs. The pictures of Fleabag are the copyright of Eddie Minnis and used with permission. The cartoon by Stanley Burnside first appeared in *The Tribune* and is copyrighted and reproduced with permission. The photograph of Jean Knowles's potcake, Mikhail, was taken by Val Albury and is reproduced with permission. The picture of "Nellie" is reproduced with permission of David Cates, the President of the Bahamas Historical Society. Other pictures of dogs were taken by WF and MI.

We are grateful to Lawrence Erlbaum Associates for permission to utilize information from our paper published in the *Journal of Applied Animal Welfare Science*, the editor of *Anthrozoös*, Anthony Podberscek, for permission to use information here from our papers published in that journal, and for permission from Marie Sairsingh-Mills, editor of the *Research Journal of The College Of The Bahamas* to include material which first appeared in that journal. We are also indebted to Neil Sealy for agreeing to publish our first articles on roaming dogs.

Foreword: The Bahamian Perspective

As the Minister responsible for the Dog Licence Act and the national animal control program, I am well aware of the size and scope of the issues relating to animal welfare and control and the efforts made over the years to manage these problems.

As the authors point out, The Bahamas is not alone, either in the Caribbean or elsewhere, in having a pet over-population problem. Since 1998, we have been making the first systematic study of dog ownership in the Caribbean which allows the issues surrounding dog ownership to be placed in a cultural context relevant to the small island states of the Region. In this way, it is possible to consider dog ownership not using cultural norms from Western Europe or North America but our own.

Using historical reports to place the association of man and dog in a long-term Bahamian setting, the reaction of society and government to the continual irritant of roaming dogs can be seen back to the 1850s. The fact that Bahamians have lived with roaming "potcakes" so long has resulted in many thinking that there is little which can be done but accept roaming dogs as part of the Bahamian landscape. However, others think otherwise and the concern of society for pets has resulted in legislations specifically designed to protect animals and the establishment of a number of organizations connected with dog welfare.

As much as we love potcakes as pets, the presence of any type of dog roaming the streets is unacceptable. This publication dispels some of the myths concerning roaming dogs and dog ownership, particularly as they relate to potcakes, so that we are able to address dog welfare in a systematic fashion. Unless we ask the right questions and appreciate the problems fully, we cannot implement policies which will improve the welfare of dogs.

By addressing dog welfare issues, this book also makes an important contribution to The Bahamas' submission to the United Nations on biodiversity and is a major contribution to the invasive species project of the Bahamas Environment, Science and Technology Commission.

I hope that this book will be read by pet lovers, policy makers and educators as well as students of The Bahamas, because as the authors show, pet ownership impinges upon many aspects of our lives. It is clear that we, as humans have much to gain by strengthening our ties with "man's best friend"—dogs.

—*V. Alfred Gray*
Minister of Agriculture, Fisheries
and Local Government
Nassau, The Bahamas

Foreword: The Human-Animal Bond

Dogs began sharing human settlements almost as soon as people built them. Today, throughout the world, dogs are one of the more common city dwellers. Despite their pervasiveness and the importance of dogs to human society, there are few careful, objective studies of dog-human interactions in the urban setting. While there are many similarities among cities, including their peoples and their dogs, there are also important differences. The environment, history, and culture of the people in the city make for interesting differences from city to city; these differences also make for interesting variations in the relationship that city dwellers have with their dogs, both owned pets and those roaming free.

Humans and their activities are the most important parts of the dog environment. The study of the dog has to be more than a study of local weather conditions and natural resources. The ecology of the urban dog includes human social views and their attitudes towards dogs, human history and politics, and human and animal public health.

The people of The Bahamas have dogs, like most peoples, but the local breed, the potcake, shares the human settings as both a pet and part of wildlife—sometimes loved, sometimes despised. The study of potcakes in New Providence is an exemplar of how to study a unique dog population. It uses observation, public records, interviews, surveys, and understandable statistics to help us understand the fascinating and complex relationship people have with their commensal canid.

At a time when developed societies appear to be concerned for the downtrodden among both people and animals, it appears that The Bahamas may have forgotten a large dog population in need of the protection enjoyed by almost all other dog breeds. This book, besides being a careful ecological study, is also a cry for help for a suffering animal population. The book asks for a reevaluation of the people and their relationship with their potcakes. The demographic and public health data, carefully analyzed, argues that it is time to appreciate these docile and loyal dogs for what they are—animals to be enjoyed that are worthy of our concern and care. But this can only happen when the people of The Bahamas—indeed all of us—recognize that whatever happens to dogs has less to do with the biology of the dogs and more to with the values, attitudes, and politics of humans.

—Alan M. Beck
School of Veterinary Medicine
Purdue University

The Potcake in Me

Marion Bethel

I am whatever you want me to be

the mongrel child at the city dump
foraging for potcake of green peas and rice
and pineappled ham skin two days after Xmas

a woman of three or more babyfathers
impervious to your treats of sterilisation
deaf to offerings of safe birth control

the young man cupping his crotch squeezing
in between binges of beer before proving
the violence and power of his phallic imagination

a girl in uniform skipping to the tightrope
of a feverish man of business during schooltime
adding to her chest and ankle a bounty of gold chains

the human puppy in a bucket still attached
to a pulsing placenta determined
to live beyond the drama of sperm and egg

a pack of stray barefoot boys forepaws
raised expectantly for small change roaming
sniffing the parking lots for fastfood bones

but most of all I am your shadow

the multiplication of all your fears
fastened to your heel or backside
the dark figure in which you hide

your anger insecurity your self-hatred
all that you reject and can't accept
you palt me with rocks and stones

I dog your bogus love
With my public sex unashamed
peppering your thoughts your groin

like crushed bird peppers red hot bullets
increasing the pitch of your fantasy
and you scald me with boiling water

I shadow your counterfeit love
with my public desire to love you
and be adored by you

I dog your steps catching all your hell
holding all the pain and scars wounds
refuse you refuse to face to survive

whatever I am I have been with you

since the beginning of time
I am your story your mangy history
Your fleabitten language and tongue

Your tick infested culture your life
…and Fleaby begat Brokeleg begat
One-eye begat Nugget begat Blackie

begat Pinky begat Threeleg begat
Bad Blood begat Sea-Egg begat High Yaller
begat Fleajangles begat Peanut begat…

I am also the subdued patch of shade

waiting at your heels conscious
of your desires your longings sheltering
you from heat and the glare of unwanted light

carrying for you the love and compassion
that are you when you choose to know it
I am your protector shadow

I have no where to go

Potcakes

1

New Providence

Good heavens! who could not look upon the scene before me, the ocean covered over with light and of a thousand radiant hues—the heavens all in a glow—the moon beaming forth a splendour quite indescribable—the fragrance of a thousand wild flowers filling the air—the leaves of the trees gently responding to the kisses of the light winds—the waves of the sea rolling in majesty at my feet—the breakers at a distance seen like rising mountains of snow, often assuming the most fantastic shapes, but lingering long enough in their foaming whiteness to catch the brilliant hues of the moon-beams as they break over them, and feel the glow of inspiration...[1]

New Providence, one of hundreds of islands that comprise The Bahamas, is the site of the Bahamian capital, Nassau. In 2000, it was home to 210,832 people (69% of the nation's population) in 59,712 households.[2] With a land area of about 200 square kilometres,[3] the island is densely populated with over 1,000 persons per square kilometre.

Nassau was formally also the British colonial capital,[4] and its colonial past can still be seen in the city's buildings. Slaves were brought directly from Africa and also indirectly by American Loyalists in the 1780s; slaves accompanying Loyalists more than doubled the population of Nassau.[5] After the abolition of slavery, slaves captured in transit to other countries were sometimes settled in the then outlying settlements of New Providence.[6] Thus, even after the end of slavery under British rule, people of African and other origins settled in the island.[7] By the 1860s the "chief ingredients" of the racial mix of The Bahamas were in place.[8] In more recent years, the economic opportunities of the islands have attracted nationals from the West Indies and beyond, as well as economic refugees, mainly from Haiti.[9] Currently about 13% of the population are non-Bahamian.[10]

1

Historically, it would seem that The Bahamas was not deemed to be of much strategic importance and has been considered a "backwater" or "marginal" colony.[11] Over the years, Nassau has experienced a series of economic boom and bust cycles, caused by both internal and external shocks, and it had to wait until the latter part of the twentieth century before achieving sustained economic growth, primarily based on tourism.[12]

Given its proximity to North America, and its paradise image, The Bahamas and New Providence have been attractive to tourists. The first tourists started to arrive in the 1740s[13] and "winter residents" came as far back as 1898.[14] Thus, Bahamians have been in close contact with foreigners for many years, particularly after the expansion of tourism in the 1950s,[15] and exposed to their expectations and aspirations. Tourism is predominantly associated with the north and west of the island, and it is there that its effects are most evident. Since the 1970s, the interaction between Bahamians and foreigners has increased with the ever-greater influence of television (both satellite and cable) and the cinema.

Tourism is now the single biggest industry in the country and in 2000 close to 4.3 million visitors came to The Bahamas and tourism earned the country $1.8 billion.[16] Thus, The Bahamas is a very public place, seen by over 14 times as many visitors as residents, so the behaviour of residents in tourist areas can have considerable economic impact upon the well-being of the economy[17] and tourism in particular.[18]

Today, the bulk of the population continues to live in Nassau itself, which is located in the northeastern part of New Providence. The population is expanding to the south of central Nassau (South Beach) and subdivisions are being developed also to the west of Nassau. To the south of the old city centre are still remnants of slave or "coloured" areas and these "over-the-hill" communities (Bain Town, Grant's Town etc.) continue to be considered the poorer areas of the city. The more northeasterly part of the island includes homes of established "old money" families, and properties along Eastern Road are much sought after. To the west of Nassau there is an extensive "hotel strip," along Cable Beach, and many homes for "snow birds" and winter residents. At the westerly tip of the island is the gated community of Lyford Cay, home to many rich and famous people. In recent years, the west has become increasingly fashionable for middle and upper class Bahamians (as well as foreigners) wishing to escape the crowds and congested roads of the eastern part of the island.

Although government departments consider all of New Providence as "urban,"[19] the west of the island is less densely populated than the east. This impression is enhanced by the presence of fresh water well fields, several lakes and swamps, and what is commonly known as the pine barrens, which consist mainly of Caribbean pine (*Pinus caribaea* var. *bahamenis*) around the international airport. However, subject to these topological barriers, construction of new homes and businesses in the west is beginning to alter the landscape, and its rural image is changing.

While there have been many outside influences on The Bahamas, from Columbus onwards, the most lasting change in the population occurred with the arrival of Africans under white colonial rule. Thus, the study of dogs in The Bahamas can be regarded as the study of dogs within a rapidly developing Afro-Caribbean society. However, it should be noted that peoples from other, usually European-related cultures, such as the British "expat" society of the 1950s and 1960s prior to independence,[20] have influenced the way Bahamians treat animals, particularly during the twentieth century.

2

Dogs in New Providence

[At] night armies of dogs begin to chase passing cars
being driven through side streets of New Providence.[1]

Dogs appear to have been on the island for hundreds of years, as Christopher Columbus reported seeing a mute type of dog when he first arrived in 1492.[2] Juan La Costa says that dogs in St. Domingo "were made pets and fattened for eating."[3] If this is so, that would suggest that dogs were kept for purposes similar to those elsewhere.[4] The Lucayans, the original inhabitants of the islands, who may have had similar customs throughout the region, clearly loved their dogs:

> At first there were no dogs at St. Domingo but a small mute creature resembling a
> dog, with a nose like that of a fox, which the natives call "aco." The Indians were so
> fond of these little animals that they carried them on their shoulders wherever they
> went, or nourished them in their bosoms.[5]

This description has been considered as being applicable also to The Bahamas.[6] In 1493, Columbus brought dogs with him to the Antilles.[7] So European dogs were introduced to the West Indies soon after Columbus discovered the islands. The indigenous dogs, augmented and bred by Spanish and/or Bermudian and English imports, may have persisted,[8] despite the demise of the indigenous Lucayans themselves, some of whom may have been killed by Spanish dogs,[9] and the subsequent influx of settlers and invaders from Africa, Europe and North America.

An early record of dogs in Nassau is in a picture. Woodes Rogers, first Royal Governor (1718–1721 and 1729–1732), was painted receiving seals of office and the picture includes a spaniel next to his wife.[10] Thus, at least in wealthy households, dogs were pets and sufficiently prized to be included in important portraits. (It seems that the indigenous dogs have had to wait until the twentieth century to be painted.[11])

Mark Catesby, who visited The Bahamas in the 1720s, observed that the country "was deficient of the numbers and variety of animals . . . except a few beasts of use that have been introduced there (such as, horses, cows, sheep, goats, hogs and dogs)."[12] This statement may allow us to infer that dogs were at least not uncommon in the early half of the eighteenth century. It also indicates that there were already introduced dogs of different breeds in Nassau, or at least many different looking dogs.

A street name, "Dog Flea Alley," probably laid out after 1768,[13] may indicate the presence of poorly kept dogs on the then southeastern outskirts of Nassau. In the 1780s, a visitor complained that the "greatest inconvenience there has been is from the plague of numerous vermin, or insects, which torment . . . both night and day."[14] This account, which lists many "vermin," omits any mention of dogs, and so it would seem they were not a nuisance at that time.

A "tax upon the keepers of all dogs within certain limits of this island of New Providence" was proposed in 1802,[15] probably as a revenue-raising measure. By the end of 1803, when the law was in force, it was said that "this tax appears to be very unproductive . . . very few returns have been made."[16] So it appears that the tax may have been unpopular and that owners did not pay it, possibly due to poor enforcement—which continues with the current dog license. This disregard for taxes on dogs may be the origin for the subsequent unwillingness of owners to license their dogs, which has persisted to the present day.

In the early 1820s, Nassau was said to be a quiet place, as "There is no noise or disturbance in the streets in the evenings."[17] This might suggest that barking dogs were not that common, at least in the higher-class areas.[18] In 1830, the tax on male dogs was £1 ($85 at today's value) and for female dogs £3[19] ($255 at today's value) belonging to owners living between Fort Montague, Fort Charlotte and the Blue Hills[20]; so only the wealthy would be able to own dogs in the city area. (Until 1826, slaves were not legally allowed to own property,[21] so presumably such taxes would have only been payable by a small number of people, even if slaves had dogs.) Even at this time, lost puppies, of no specific breed ("a yellow puppy with white legs, ears and tail cropped very close"[22]) were clearly valued and warranted the offer of a suitable reward if found.

The first official admission of a "stray dog problem" appears to be that in the Statute Laws of The Bahamas of 1841. In that year it was noted that

> Whereas the great increase of Dogs in the Colony has, in many instances, become a nuisance, and it would tend to abate such nuisance, were a moderate Tax imposed on Dogs kept within the Town and Suburbs of Nassau, and within the limits of other Towns.[23]

This law imposed a tax of four shillings and two pence a year (about $18 at today's prices) on all dogs owned in central Nassau and as far south as Grant's Town. It is clear that the purpose of this tax was to curb the dog population within the city. However, poorer people, many of whom would have been people of African origin or ex-slaves, lived in Grant's Town.[24] These inhabitants would, presumably, have been prevented from legally owning dogs due to the tax, which would have been expensive for them, as many ex-slaves received little money as part of their wages (for example, 25 cents a week in one case, or $1 a month in another in the late 1830s[25] or about four shillings a month.[26]) Thus the size of the tax, together with possibly lax enforcement, may have resulted in widespread non-compliance with the tax.

In 1849, Henry Fleeming was fined 10 shillings (about $48 at today's value) "for setting his dog upon James Moss, to put him in fear."[27] This report shows that dogs could be a real nuisance and one which society would not tolerate, at least in some instances. It also makes clear that owners were held responsible for the actions of their pets, and there were limits as to how dogs could be used.

In 1856 a dog license law was imposed on all dogs in New Providence.[28] The Act said that "the number of dogs . . . have increased to such an extent as to become a public nuisance," as if it was recognized that the previous law had failed in its stated aim to curb the dog population. In 1842, the dog population had been described only as "in many instances, become a nuisance," whereas in 1856 dogs were now a "public nuisance." The tax meant that it cost one shilling ($3.90 at today's value) for the first dog and nine pence ($2.90 at today's value) for subsequent dogs per quarter[29] (the equivalent of $15.70 and $11.80 per year respectively) to own a dog anywhere in New Providence. This would have been an attempt to further limit the number of people who could own dogs, and hence limit the dog population. The increase in the area in which dogs were taxed may also have been in recognition of owned dogs roaming into the city limits from elsewhere. Clearly, to limit the number of dogs in the city by restricting ownership within the city, as the earlier law intended, would not necessarily reduce the presence of dogs there. Dogs do not respect city limits and can have comparatively large home ranges on a small island like New Providence,[30] particularly if seeking food or mates. It seems reasonable to assume that these taxes would mean that all poorer people would be disqualified from legally having dogs. Therefore, it is easy to get the impression that lawmakers disliked having dogs in the city of Nassau, and it might be interpreted that owners outside the city were considered the cause of this "nuisance."

The 1856 Act was also forward-looking, as it also made owners responsible for the actions of their dogs,[31] an issue which reoccurs in later Acts and is still important today.

An illustration of cotton being loaded in Nassau Harbour, printed in London, (1860s) includes a roaming brown dog, apparently barking at a horse and another, also printed in London, of "The town and port of Nassau" includes a dog.[32] The first picture gives the impression of roaming dogs being a nuisance in a similar way as they are today when they bark at cars or people.

In the 1860s, considerable monetary value was placed on purebred dogs:

LOST

In the Public Market on Saturday last a liver-colored curly Retriever puppy answering to the name of "Tiger" or "Tig." Whoever will give information that will lead to the recovery of the same shall be liberally rewarded by the owner.[33]

This suggests that at least some owners were fond of their pets. Further, theft of a dog was punishable by a fine of up to six months in prison for a first offence and £20 ($1,600 at today's value) or 18 months in prison for a second offence.[34]

In addition, there was an unpopular import tax of 10 shillings ($41 at today's value) per dog.[35] (The current charge for an import permit is $10 per dog.) This tax would have the effect of deterring people from importing dogs and increasing the value of dogs, presumably pure-bred dogs bred locally. This would mean that poorer people would be unlikely to be able to buy pure-bred dogs.

Despite the laws, in the 1870s Charles Ives gives the feeling that dogs were common and possibly also neglected:

That pet of many a household—man's friend, companion, guard and protector—the much abused dog—is not only frequently met with upon the islands.[36]

He considered the "mild and soothing air" as the reason why the dogs "are too lazy and indolent to bark" (referring to the mute dogs which Columbus saw) but later he stated that the dogs were "too amiable" to bark.[37] He makes it clear that roosters made more noise than the dogs. However, this contest as to which animal made most noise at night may have been very close; William Drysdale, writing in the early 1880s, indicates that his cook's dog "is a cur of the currest kind, black and gray, but an affectionate little rascal and a good watch-dog, for he barks at night on the smallest provocation."[38]

However, the law failed to curb dog ownership, or at least the dog population. A tourist who wanted to buy a dog was told "Everybody in Nassau has a dog, and they all bark all night," and "stray" dogs and puppies could be found at tourist sites.[39] Drysdale gives the clear impression that the local dogs were common and that they certainly did bark, at least at night. However, a law of 1873 suggested that dogs were a worry to residents because owners who allowed "to be at large any unmuzzled ferocious dog or sets or urges any dog on other animal to attack, worry, or put in fear any person or animal"[40] were liable to a fine of up to 50 shillings ($172 at today's value) or 20 days in jail.

Thus despite the law, rich and poor people continued to own dogs, and the nuisance of free roaming dogs was reported in detail by a colonial judge, L. D. Powles:

The origin of the extraordinary collection of mongrels that inhabit this city and its suburbs and pass for dogs must ever remain a puzzle. Mr. Drysdale says they are "the most fearful and wonderful productions of nature."[41] Like the majority of living things in Nassau they are half-starved, and spend their nights wandering about the wealthier parts of the city, trying to pick-up scraps. Their howlings, and the crowing of the cocks, who invariably commence at 11 p.m., and continue for several hours without ceasing, make nights hideous. Some time ago a dog tax was imposed by the Legislature, but it became so unpopular, and so extremely difficult to collect that it had to be ignominiously abandoned. Wherever you go in coloured settlements, dogs run out every minute to bark at you, but I never heard of their biting anyone, and they run away if you merely turn and look at them. [42]

The malnourished appearance of the dogs had also been reported by Drysdale, and this may have been due to the high cost and scarcity of dog food.[43] Powles' classic account of the local mongrels gives us a graphic description of their characteristics, which are still seen in many dogs in the Bahamas. It confirms Ives' report of the noise due to chickens and dogs each night and it also points to society's reluctance to impose a law designed to curb the number of dogs.

In the 1890s, roaming dogs appear to have been a nuisance to everyone, and those who would have lived in upper-class areas appear to be exasperated with the situation:

As for the dogs, if Nassau has ever been more over-run than now with homeless curs that make night hideous, well, I pity those who preceded us as residents in this charming little capital.[44]

Use of the word "hideous" in these two reports may not be coincidental after all. Roaming dogs continued to cause trouble, and in 1898 it was reported that

after the hours of darkness set in a number of worthless curs congregate in the city, and commit depredations upon poultry and create nuisances which are extremely annoying.[45]

This passage may explain why the dogs finally appear to have won the competition with the poultry for making most noise at night. Dogs still roamed the streets in search of food: ". . . a dog dashed pasted us after something he saw on the pavement. It was a big piece of meat."[46]

George Northcroft's observation that "The Bahamian dog of today is neither mute, fat or loveable"[47] reiterates the impression of barking dogs which were thin and possibly sick (i.e. not "loveable") and mongrels. A photograph of Bay Street at the turn of the nineteenth century shows a dog that could easily be roaming, even if owned.[48] In poorer parts of Nassau, dogs are seen in photographs of "liberated African settlements" from (possibly) 1900 onwards.[49]

Residents of African ancestry maintained their African traditions and continued to speak their native languages in New Providence well into the twentieth century.[50] In addition, they practiced Obe, which has been defined as "a type of bad medicine"[51] and said "to have the power of taking or saving life, or causing or curing disease, of bringing ruin or creating prosperity, of discovering evil-doers or vindicating the innocent."[52] In the 1760s and again in the 1890s,[53] it was reported that dog's teeth were used in Obeah nostrums, so dogs' teeth were presumably linked with some power, or spirit attributed to dogs. This could have included fecundity or other characteristics. Thus, dogs would have had a purpose, albeit limited, beyond that of food, companion or guardian.

Dogs were included in an act of 1895 to consolidate duties on imports, and in 1898, another law was passed that required owners to license dogs.[54] Presumably this was yet another attempt to limit dog ownership, and of course it would allow owners of dogs to be identified. However, in 1900 that measure seems to have had little effect, and it was "reenacted" and revised in 1942.[55] It then cost five shillings ($11.60 at today's value) a year to license a dog or spayed female and ten shillings ($23.25 at today's value) a year for an intact female.[56] These fees would have been substantial when one considers that the daily wage was four shillings for "a common labourer" in the late 1940s.[57] (The current dog license fees are $2 for a male or spayed female and $6 for an intact female. To put this in context, the minimum weekly wage is $150.[58]) The size of the fees current in the 1940s might have deterred many owners from licensing their dogs.

The debate, in 1942, clearly focused on the need to identify owners and to control the roaming of dogs,[59] an issue which seems to echo the problems suggested in the 1841 Act. The 1942 legislation appears to have been driven by the realization that winter residents and those living in upper-class areas found the sight of roaming dogs disagreeable. Such residents would not only contribute to the economy of the country, but also they would probably be influential in getting such an act passed. This new legislation made it an offence for dogs to roam at night. It is also an early example of the concern government had about the possible detrimental effect of roaming dogs on tourists. (These concerns persist[60] and are dealt with in Chapter 9.) However, this attempt to control the nuisance of roaming "curs" and their barking at night was ineffectual due to the lack of dogcatchers.[61] Irrespective of their effect on tourists, it was considered that "This uncontrolled pest [roaming dog] is very damaging to Nassau's reputation as a quiet city . . . [and a] . . . blot on the civilization of the island."[62] Later, in 1965, when dogcatchers were at work, the public wanted higher dog license fees and better law enforcement.[63]

Not all roaming dogs in the 1940s were poorly kept or unowned. A "cream coloured" dog of no specified breed had been found which "appears to have been well cared for,"[64] so while press reports focussed on thin dogs, dogs were not always neglected.

Despite these laws, packs of dogs were seen in the 1930s in Nassau (for example, 80 on Montague Beach) which were "mostly strays"[65]; a comment suggesting that some owned dogs might have been impounded. Although many "curs" were caught at various times, dogs are still seen in the same areas (for example, Shirley Street, the hospital area, Parliament Street) to this day.[66] Complaints about free-roaming dogs are a recurring feature in the letters pages of the national newspapers[67] and the subject of numerous editorials. In fact, one newspaper went so far as to suggest that motorists did the community a favour by knocking down roaming dogs. However, this recommendation is now a source of embarrassment,[68] and residents are now given advice as to what to do should their car hit a dog.[69] This issue shows how attitudes towards roaming dogs have changed in recent years.

Recently, it has been claimed that many people have obtained dogs to guard their homes in response to an increase in crime,[70] but due to poor confinement, these animals joined the roaming population.[71] (The use of dogs to protect homes is considered later.) This lack of control probably explains why complaints about free-roaming dogs continue to this day, with the usual issues of "what is government going to do"[72] being countered by accusations that owners are to blame for the "problem" due to "irresponsible" pet ownership.[73] The frustration of some residents with "stray" dogs can be illustrated by the demand that all dogs be neutered.[74] Sometimes, however, it is made clear that both sides must work together to reduce the roaming dog population.[75] Such exchanges between the public and government officials typically occur in the aftermath of an attack by dogs on residents or visitors or reports of a perceived public health threat associated with dogs.[76]

Since the 1980s, issues associated with dogs have taken a new twist. "Image" dogs, such as pit bulls and rottweilers etc., started to become popular and command high prices.[77] There has been a rise in the number of companies offering "attack" or guard dog services. Since 1991, dogs have reportedly killed three people; the last attack was by free-roaming dogs. Two of the deaths were caused by pit bulls, but the type responsible for the last death is still unknown. This has focused attention on the historical as well as more recent issues concerning dog ownership, and made people realize that dogs can be a real threat to society, rather than merely a "nuisance." The fact that pit bulls are probably the most popular type on the island, together with the inability of some owners to confine their pets, means that society must expect these animals to roam (which they do[78]) and breed with other dogs, with unknown effects on the behaviour of the roaming population. However, reports that "vicious dogs," such as pit bulls, will make other dogs vicious may be exaggerated due to the inheritability of their "breed" associated traits.[79] (Dog bites and deaths caused by dogs are considered in more detail in Chapter 16.)

Recent bad publicity about dogs has occurred against a backdrop of continual fears concerning rabies and other public health issues related to dogs.[80] No case of rabies has been reported in The Bahamas.[81] However, its proximity to countries with rabies, and its many ports of entry, in particular by sea, make the importation of this disease by dogs a possibility.[82] The risk has been much aired in the media and invariably used to worry people about roaming dogs. This has resulted in many people considering free-roaming dogs as not only a nuisance but also as a health hazard. Sadly, adverse publicity about dogs results in an increase in the number of acts of cruelty towards animals.[83]

In 1822, England passed the first law to prevent cruelty to animals.[84] The Bahamas followed this lead, and in 1841 passed a law concerning animal cruelty[85]; although dogs were not specifically mentioned, they would probably have been covered.[86] However, it was not until 1892 that a society for the prevention of cruelty to animals was formed at the instigation of church leaders in response to "a great deal which can only rightly be described as positive cruelty [to animals]."[87] The formation of this society was surrounded by a number of letters of support[88] and the Governor chaired the inaugural meeting. By 1908, that society had failed, and "Our Dumb Friends League" was founded; amongst other things, this group organized the "humane destruction of dogs." By 1924, with the League no longer operating, the wife of a colonial official started what is now the Bahamas Humane Society.[89] This is the island's only animal "shelter." Towards the end of the twentieth century, several animal welfare organizations were formed and these have contributed to keeping the welfare of dogs, owned and unowned, in the public eye.[90] These groups have played important roles in providing neuter programmes, raising awareness of animal abuse and lobbying government for changes in the law concerning animals.

Today, dogs are found all over the island, and their distribution follows that of the human population. In the mid-1970s it was noted that "dogs are mainly concentrated among the poorer section of the community" despite the "daily dog catching efforts of the [Humane] Society."[91] Although almost all residents agree that there is a "stray dog problem," those in central Nassau[92] are most likely to have roaming dogs in their neighbourhood. We could crudely describe the socioeconomic conditions in New Providence as follows: central Nassau as poorer, the south as middle income, and the west and the east as richer.[93] In central Nassau, 80% (of 120 replies) compared with 77% (of 35 replies), 67% (of 43 replies) and 65% (of 82 replies) in the southern, western and eastern parts of the island respectively (p=0.075) reported roaming dogs. Thus it would seem that the distribution of the dog population has changed little in 25 years and that roaming dogs are still most common in poorer areas. These figures do not reflect the regional variation in the number of owned dogs per household, from 1.67 (se=0.254) in the eastern, 1.16 (se=0.189) in the central, and 1.44 (se=0.371) in the western to 0.57 (se=0.698) in the southern areas (p=0.025) of New Providence. However, these figures probably reflect socioeconomic variability associated with these areas.

Thus, although dogs, owned and roaming, are found islandwide, there are regional variations. It should be noted that the nuisance of roaming dogs is not confined to any particular area or social or economic group.[94] Our studies have not examined the detailed differences between neighbourhoods, as we have tried to get an overall impression of dog ownership by Bahamians. However, we are aware of variations within the island and where appropriate we refer to a small-scale study, made by students at The College of The Bahamas, in Bain Town (an established, poorer community in south-central Nassau) and Yamacraw (a newer, middle-class subdivision to the east of Nassau[95]).

This brief overview of dogs in New Providence shows that they have always been part of The Bahamian household from the time of the Lucayans onwards and their treatment has varied according to customs of the time. The arrival of people of African origin and other immigrants probably increased the number of dog owners, despite the efforts of laws to limit dog ownership. Probably, as the human population increased and New Providence became more urban, society, under the influence of foreign views of pet welfare, implemented more rules to govern dog ownership. However, these regulations concerning dog ownership have not prevented many owners from allowing their pets to annoy neighbours and visitors. As the human population lives in an increasingly dense urban environment, there seems to be less tolerance to roaming dogs. These worries appear to have polarized owners on one hand and non-dog owners and government officials on the other about the actions required to stop dogs being a nuisance to society. Typically the issues become topical when dog attacks are publicized, but rarely for long. Reasons for dog ownership may have changed little since the time of the Lucayans—although dogs are no longer eaten—but security concerns and the financial benefits of breeding selected dog types appear to have driven modern owners to seek image dogs, with biting histories, in preference to local mongrels (see chapters 10, 11, and 12 below). This change has introduced a new dimension to the dog population, the results of which we are yet to fully appreciate.

3

Potcakes

Potcakes . . . have a mild temperament and are generally considered loveable and loyal.[1]

Potcake: burnt or very crisp food adhering to the cooking vessel, considered a delicacy.[2]

Potcake: any mongrel dog of no definable breed.

Short haired, light brown dog of mixed breed which is very common in The Bahamas.[3]

The local mongrels, those "most fearful and wonderful productions of nature" of Mr. Drysdale, are called potcakes.[4] The only other country where dogs are called potcakes is in the Turks and Caicos Islands, where there is now a "Potcake Foundation."[5] In fact, "potcake" appears to be a locally coined word, as it is absent from dictionaries[6] outside of the Caribbean. Potcakes are said to get their name from the burnt or caked food from the bottom of the family pot which was fed to them[7]; the practice of feeding dogs leftovers from household food continues to this day. Despite the commonly held belief about the origin of potcake for the indigenous dog, the *Dictionary of Bahamian English* does not commit itself on this point, unlike the *Dictionary of Caribbean English Usage*.[8] The fact that dogs eat potcake means that potcake dogs are, possibly, the only "true" Bahamians left, according to one definition of "true Bahamian."[9] In the Turks and Caicos Islands, potcakes are reported to only eat cooked food.[10] This choice might have resulted from their being fed cooked food from an early age, when taste preferences are formed,[11] which reinforces the dependency between potcakes and humans.

So far, we have been only able to trace this name for mongrel dogs back to the 1870s via oral tradition,[12] and 1970 in print,[13] although veterinarians used the word to describe a "specific type of dog" on health certificates in the 1960s.[14] In 1973, a newspaper reported a story from 1952 which referred to a "potcake dog."[15] This story is consistent with the notion that "potcake" may have been used by people of African descent well before its appearance in print. Prior to the 1970s, newspapers and books typically referred to roaming dogs (almost certainly potcakes) as mongrels or curs. Not even Powles, who was interested in Bahamian dialect, uses the word in his description of what were most certainly potcakes in the 1880s. In the 1960s, "cur" was an extremely derogatory term and was not suitable for use in Parliament.[16] This suggests that "potcake" was not used by the ruling classes and that it might have been considered a slang word and unsuitable for use in newspapers.

There is no consistent usage of the term "potcake." For most residents, it refers to *any* mongrel dog that cannot be clearly related to a breed, although the dictionary definition attributes specific characteristics to potcakes.[17] When psychology students[18] at The College of The Bahamas were asked what they understood by the word "potcake," 68% (of 37 replies) specifically stated that it referred to dogs of mixed breed; in other responses it was implied. They also considered potcakes to live on the streets and so were often unloved or without an owner. One student described a potcake as

> a resilient hound dog that lives on the streets of New Providence and other islands in The Bahamas. The potcake has become infamous for its unusual taste for garbage and [is] feared for their [sic] aggressive behaviour when in groups! Yet it is loved by many Bahamians and is a proud symbol of Bahamian culture. The potcake can be bred with any other dog and most of the time they are crossbreeds. Its short hair allows the potcake to survive the high humidity levels in The Bahamas. They also have a heightened sense of intuition as they make good guard dogs.

This mixed response to potcakes—icon and fallen pet—is repeated in our other interviews.

The description of one potcake, "Chelsea," could apply to a great many:

> She has floppy ears, skinny legs and a bunch of colours in her short hair including black, white and brown. Her father is unknown. . . . The moniker [of potcake] reflects a mingled and untraceable heritage. . . . They [potcakes] wear their hearts in their eyes, right where you can see them. There are no hidden agendas or deceptive tactics.[19]

The Bahamas Kennel Club has defined the potcake as having distinct characteristics. Its standard is as follows:

GENERAL DESCRIPTION

The Bahamian Potcake is a medium size dog standing 18–22" [45–55cm] (Bitches), 20–24" [50–60cm] (Dogs), at the shoulder with moderate bone and substance. Approximate level back, alert expression, swift and agile movement, somewhat leery of strangers, but a good household companion. Approx. weight 34–40 lbs [15.4–18.1kg] (Bitches), 40–45 lbs [18.1–20.3kg] (Dogs).

HEAD

The head is characterized by a moderately wide backskull, slight stop with somewhat narrow muzzle (not pointed) which is only slightly shorter than the backskull. A clean, smooth face. The teeth in a scissors bite, and the relatively large ears tend more to the rose shape but are very mobile. The medium size eyes are dark to hazel. Nose, preferably black.

NECK AND SHOULDERS

The neck is moderately long with slight arch at the nape and tapers to smooth fitting, well laid back shoulders, strong and lean.

BODY

The chest is moderately long, the ribs reaching about to the elbow, and extending rather well back. The tuck-up, though apparent, is not too pronounced and the loin muscles are strong and slightly arched, though the topline is essentially level. The loin is not too long and the dog is slightly longer than high, measured from point of forechest to point of rump.

LEGS AND FEET

The legs are straight, moderately boned with the elbow set directly below the peak of the shoulder. The feet are tight and firm, well padded with high arched toes. The hind legs are somewhat angulated at both stifle and hock, with the femur and tibia being near the same length. When standing, the feet toe neither in nor out.

TAIL

The tail is set neither high not low, reaching about to the hock, well covered but not heavy. Broad at base and tapering to end. The hair slightly longer on the underside. When the dog is moving, the tail may be carried straight but often over towards the back.

COAT

The coat is short, close and neither silky nor coarse.

COLOUR AND MARKINGS

Shades of brown going from tan to light brown. Black (all these colours may have a white flash on chest and/or toes), black and tan, brindle, white with large black or brown markings.

MOVEMENT

The movement is free, easy, graceful and with a spring in the step. There is good reach in front and decided in the rear. Going away, the legs will tend to converge as the dog's speed increases.

SUMMARY

The Bahamian Potcake should be a healthy, hardy dog that could survive and thrive in the underbrush and rocky terrain of the Bahamian Islands. He is a good watch dog and household companion."[20]

Although the term "pure-bred potcake"[21] is sometimes used, we consider this to
be (at least now) an oxymoron. Due to the interbreeding of what some might term the
traditional potcake with pure-bred dogs, some claim that "real" potcakes are rare. The
popular perception, as expressed by the students above, is that the potcake is a mongrel,
so this is the usage that we have adopted here. Some people distinguish between a
"cross-bred"—a mongrel that has recognizable characteristics of a pure-bred dog—and
a potcake to differentiate a potcake from a mongrel that is still closely related to a
breed.[22] From our pictures of potcakes, it is clear that potcakes, as commonly perceived, do not look alike. This probably means that they result from some level of human intervention, as the pictures suggest no obvious selection to the mean, which
would be expected if environmental conditions were responsible for selection.[23] If that
were the case, there would be little variation in the appearance of potcakes. This observation confirms the interaction between potcakes and humans, a theme that recurs
throughout our studies.

"Potcake" is used in contexts wider than the dictionary suggests, as the word has
many meanings and associations. Responses which potcakes invoke include:

> I had prejudged them as insignificant. . . . After all, they were considered to be low
> bred; they ate out of the garbage; they lived outside amidst the elements and "we
> only knew them when we needed them."[24]

> They are practically rejects in elitist circles in spite of their prowess, agility, fearless-
> ness and resilience. There is a total disregard for their diligence, loyalty and willing-
> ness to die to protect their boundaries. Even so, not many potcakes experience the
> comfort of a warm place to sleep or three square meals, fed to them by the hands of
> a caring master.[25]

It also has a social meaning that is summed up by such phrases as "shepherd-
potcake mentality" or even "potcake culture."[26] German shepherd dogs, like other
pure-bred dogs, are expensive and so more likely to belong to the rich. Potcakes are
cheap, or indeed worthless,[27] and so the poor can own them. Thus, "Shepherd-
potcake" mentality is a way of attributing differences between rich and poor people.
This expression also encompasses aspects of the "haves" and "have-nots," as potcakes
are regarded as getting less care (particularly health care) than pure-bred dogs. "Potcake culture" has been used as a synonym for "backward," "uneducated," "aesthetically
displeasing" or something that is not "elitist." The term "potcake dogs," when applied
to people, indicates that they are disliked, either because of the way they look or act.[28]
Again, when used to refer to a person, the term can also mean "reject" or someone who
does not belong to a particular group.[29] "Potcake" is also used as a pen name on a Bahamian youth Internet site in which uncomplimentary exchanges are made.[30]

A potcake was also a character in a newspaper cartoon. Cartoons by Eddie Minnis appeared in the *Tribune* and his record covers featured a potcake called Fleabag,[31]
"affectionately known as Fleabs."[32] Fleabag was "Granny's" constant companion and
confidant.[33] She clearly loved the dog, and the dog was most possessive of Granny; he

was truly a companionable animal. The potcake's name (and the pictures) suggests that Granny's dog was sick (at least suffered from fleas), so why did Granny not get him treated? Was she unwilling to spend money on Fleabag because he was a potcake? Even if the animal was not sick, the name suggests an animal to which Granny gave little care, despite the role it played in her life. Although Fleabag has no obvious fleas[34] in more recent cartoons, we have been assured that he still has them; "he is a potcake after all!"[35] It should also be noted that "Fleabag" has resonance with Dog Flea Alley and reinforces the idea that potcakes are sick.

In recent years, the potcake has appeared in some popular songs.[36] The potcake has also been used by Eddie Minnis in his lyric "Mix-up dog" in a homosexual context. The mix-up dog is considered "stray" in that "anytime he see another male . . . he want to start to romance."[37] Thus through a series of puns, Minnis uses the potcake, "Mix-up dog," who "tink he got pedigree" as a vehicle to raise the issue of homosexuality in a society which discriminates against such behaviour.[38]

Potcake has explicitly entered pop culture through at least two songs: "The Cry of the Potcake" from the CD *Down Home*,[39] sung by Phil Stubbs; and "Who will love the potcake?" by Joy DiAntonio, and sung by Lovey Forbes[40] from The Turks and Caicos. The rhetorical nature of the latter title indicates that there is little love for the potcake in The Turks and Caicos Islands. The words of these songs indicate the popular image of the canine potcake. In the insert notes to *Down Home*, Stubbs writes:

> "Pot-cake" is a local breed of dogs indigenous to The Bahamas. I was inspired to write this song based on poor treatment they receive in our society as opposed to dogs with pedigree.

The words of Stubbs' song, made more powerful by using the first person singular, resonate with our observations concerning owned dogs. The song describes a potcake who faithfully guards his owner's yard but is barely fed or watered in return.[41] The potcake describes his increasing neglect as he grew up[42] and how he now roams the streets knocking over garbage bins and getting into fights. He looks enviously at purebred dogs and wishes he got the care they received. He laments his infestation of fleas and worries that if he gets mangy he will be taken to the shelter and be put down. The line preceding the final chorus adds a poignancy which suggests despair:

> Somebody help me.
> [Chorus]
> They don't love me;
> They only know me when they need me.

The references to mange and fleas again pick up the idea that owned potcakes are unhealthy, as depicted by Minnis. The song also refers to an attempt to confine the dog, which, although a failure, does show that the owner tried to stop the dog from roaming.

DiAntonio's lyrics:

> Who will love the potcake by the roadside?
> He's yours for free, he's not for sale

highlight the issues that recur in our studies: potcakes are worthless, at least economically, and are associated with dogs which roam.

The international hit song "Who Let the Dogs Out?" by the Bahamian group Baha Men was also very popular in The Bahamas. The song, apparently concerning dogs, has sexually provocative words, and makes no actual reference to potcakes. As few people know or understand the words, beyond the chorus, the song has been adopted by several animal welfare groups in The Bahamas.[43] In a country with many roaming dogs, the question "Who let the dogs out?" is an important one, particularly as it relates to dogs. In addition to these "popular" references to potcakes, they also appear in more "serious" poetry.[44]

The long relationship that residents have with dogs, and in particular potcakes, has resulted in anthropomorphism of potcakes, and identification with their actions by humans.[45] "Potcake," as applied to a male, suggests a lack of commitment to a relationship; applied to a female, it denotes that the woman has a questionable upbringing, or comes from a poor family, or may even be "loose." Sexual connotations were also applied to Stubbs' song, with "potcake" being a euphemism for a man and the song being a coded story about human relationships.[46] There may even be a subconscious empathy with potcakes, as they, like humans, participate in relationships of convenience[47] and are exposed to female-dominated rearing. This empathy may arise in both formal and informal human relationships, as males are sometimes absent from the household and may indulge in "sweet-hearting."[48]

Outspoken critics of Bahamian society have drawn parallels between the behaviour of Bahamian males and potcakes.[49] This personification of the potcake in the context of "irresponsible [sexual] behaviour" is unfortunate, as it reinforces the negative image of the potcake. Further, male sexual connotations with "potcake" can be found on an Internet site that advertises potency potions and uses "potcake" as slang for "penis."[50] This usage suggests that the potcake is seen as an irresponsible, virile animal (as possibly alluded to in the quotation on page 18 above,[51] but also to be emulated or envied. This could be associated with the fact that puppies are seen all year round, which has resulted in the commonly held (but mistaken) belief that individual potcakes breed all the time, i.e. are sexually potent, always have a mate or are virile. The sexual aspect of potcakes has been graphically illustrated in the tabloid press and is alluded to in other papers.[52]

As will become clear, the study of dog welfare in New Providence is essentially the study of the welfare of potcakes. Not only are they the most common type of dog, but they also make up almost all of the roaming dog population. Regrettably this association has resulted in high-ranking officials confusing potcakes with stray dogs and using the two terms interchangeably.[53] Thus it becomes easy for potcakes to be considered only as stray dogs.[54] This again portrays the potcake unfavourably and suggests that potcakes are unowned and given little care.

Others have likened the way mothers nurture their children to the way owners look after their potcakes; they

> keep them chained, and if they bark too much, they throw hot water on them to quiet them. When they are hungry, they feed them the junk of the kitchen. If they survive, they are valuable to invest in.[55]

Even after ignoring the hyperbole, the use of the potcake for this comparison is unfair. It paints a picture of owned potcakes as not being merely poorly treated, but being inhumanely treated, a far graver offence. As a result, it presents a distorted picture of pet ownership, which is particularly untrue of the many owners who love their potcakes and care for them unstintingly.

Potcakes make excellent pets, and this important companionable attribute has been noted in the press[56] and is recognized by residents and foreigners alike. There are many cases of tourists adopting free-roaming potcakes and having them flown to their homelands, and 41% of residents have adopted dogs or cats.[57] It has even been suggested that foreigners who have adopted potcakes might become tourists to The Bahamas, wanting to "see where their puppies come from."[58] Tourists can buy souvenirs associated with potcakes, such as soft toys and tee-shirts.[59] Potcakes are also discussed (usually superficially and/or inaccurately) in publications aimed at tourists.[60] This again reflects the ambivalence of residents towards potcakes[61]; on the one hand potcakes are considered a nuisance, but on the other they are considered "truly Bahamian," and tourists are encouraged to remember their vacation in The Bahamas through potcakes.

The fact that potcakes "are the most faithful dogs we have in Nassau," and are hardy animals[62] is contrasted with the idea that they also represent what is least desirable; a pedigree dog is seen to be superior to a mongrel just because it looks better, or has a known heritage. Additionally, ownership of a pedigree dog is another way of displaying wealth and, possibly, influence,[63] as pure-bred animals cost hundreds, if not thousands of dollars,[64] in contrast to the worthless potcake, which anyone can own. "Image" dogs may contribute to desires for power, prestige, status and influence, which dog owners have to a greater extent than cat owners.[65]

These aspects contrast with one local "character," who sells car hubcaps and delivers "anti-crime homilies." He is called "Potcake," and so proud of his alias that he is reluctant to divulge his real name.[66] Further positive associations with potcakes include using a potcake as a mascot in a school anti-drug campaign, as sniffer-dogs and by taking potcakes into schools when teaching good pet care.[67] "Peppy Potcake" appeared in a children's story which described the adventures of a potcake puppy from birth in the bush to a happy adoption via the Humane Society, and so highlighted the plight of roaming dogs.[68] Unnamed potcakes have also been featured in a rhyming children's early-age reading book.[69] Attempts to improve the image of potcakes have included renaming them "Royal Bahamian potcakes" and claiming that they are a "breed,"[70] but this "rebranding" does not seem to have been widely adopted.[71] Thus, despite the negative associations with the word "potcake," which do little to help the welfare of dogs, potcakes do get some positive press,[72] and are used to contribute to humour in the newspapers.[73]

This brief overview of potcakes highlights the mixed emotions that they generate in society. Elsewhere, potcakes would be called mongrels, mixed-breeds or "mutts." However, potcakes have a more important place in Bahamian society than these other names suggest. This difference makes the potcake unique, not necessarily in any biological sense, but because of the way society interacts with it. Potcakes should, we feel, be regarded as more than dogs. (In other cultures "Temple dogs"—also mongrels—have a status beyond that of their breeding, so potcakes are not alone in having an elevated position.) The associations that society has with potcakes are not easily unraveled, but almost certainly affect the way many people view and therefore treat them. On one hand they are companions, guardians, a "proud symbol of Bahamian culture," an icon, but on the other hand they are a nuisance. These conflicting views of mankind's relationship with dogs are not unique to The Bahamas and raise many issues regarding how humans view and treat dogs.[74]

Despite attempts by various organizations and the enactment of legislation over the years, society has failed to control the free-roaming population and contain the nuisances caused by dogs, and potcakes in particular. This has resulted in potcakes receiving a bad press at the expense of their positive attributes. Society has lived so long with potcakes that not only "from a cultural point of view we have become accustomed to seeing stray dogs around"[75] but also a culture of itself has evolved around the concept of the potcake and the term has entered into a wider modern usage. This suggests that issues surrounding potcakes have gone beyond merely being associated with canines, and into The Bahamian psyche.[76] It would appear that humans project sexual and lineage connotations onto potcakes.[77] This probably makes issues associated with containing the potcake/dog populations more than just an exercise in animal control and pet welfare. Unless animal control/care strategies are sensitive to these cultural issues,[78] programmes designed to control pet numbers may meet with resistance, which could be rooted in issues such as sexuality, identity and class.

4

Organizations Associated with Dogs

Even if you don't want to go and take an animal up that's injured, there's animal control . . . there's the Bahamas Humane Society. . . . There's so many people you can call . . .[1]

New Providence is well endowed with organizations that have responsibilities, or have elected to undertake responsibilities, towards dogs and society. Collectively, these groups help to protect society from nuisance dogs, enhance the welfare of dogs and limit the dog population through neutering programmes.

Activities of the animal shelter

The Bahamas Humane Society[2] is the oldest animal group in the country. It is the only "shelter"[3] on the island. Today, it is the largest of the five veterinary clinics. In addition to providing a full veterinary service, it runs adoption and neuter programmes. Its adoption programme is publicized via a "Pet of the Week" spot in the national press.[4] Its officers play an important role in enforcing the Penal Code[5] with regard to cruelty to animals and it has an officer in charge of education on animal welfare.

The adoption programme allows dogs and cats to be homed which have been neutered and received their vaccinations, including that for rabies, for $40. This cost is less than that for the veterinary services, so the animal itself is effectively free. In 2001, 250 dogs were adopted out, of which 4.4% were "full breed."[6]

Although the Society is no longer responsible for catching roaming dogs, it still accepts unwanted dogs and re-homes as many of them as possible. Animals that are considered suitable for adoption are also received from the Animal Control Unit rather than being killed by euthanasia.

The Society also runs a limited neutering programme. In 1998, 200 free neuters were carried out.[7] This programme is designed to help the poorest owners to get their animals neutered. A lack of funds limits the extent of this programme, and owners are encouraged to make whatever contribution they can to the cost of the operation.

In 2001, the shelter immunized 4,056 dogs and puppies, and 2,136 dogs and puppies were immunized against rabies. One thousand and ninety-eight dogs were neutered, of which 64% were spays. Typically, almost no pure-bred animals as such are seen in the shelter; usually all would be described as "mixed" breed, i.e., potcakes.

Veterinary clinics

In addition to the Bahamas Humane Society clinic, there are four other veterinary clinics.

All the clinics offer "pro bono" services for poorer pet owners. One clinic encourages its wealthier clients to pay the veterinary bills of poorer owners, allowing more health care for animals in poorer households.

At the end of 1998 and the start of 1999, a census of the five clinics was made. In the previous 12 months, 20,140 dogs and 1,218 litters were brought into the clinics. A summary of the activities of the veterinary clinics is given in Table 4.1.

Table 4.1: Number of dogs seen by veterinary clinics in New Providence in the 12 months prior circa 1999.

	Immunized for rabies	Immunized (not rabies)	Euthanized	Neutered
Adults	1,015	3,114	655	
Puppies	1,224	7,876+	436	
All dogs*	4,349*	10,990+	1,091	2,214[§]

*At least one clinic only gave records relating to the total number of cats and dogs immunized.
+ At least one clinic reported at "least figures."
§ About 30% of neuters were on male dogs.

The subtropical climate of New Providence allows diseases to persist all year round. For example, mosquitoes are present throughout the year and so dogs can contract heart worm (*Dirofilariasis*) at any time. Other parasites of dogs include *Rhipicephalus sanguineus, Sarcoptes scabei* var. *canis, Ctenocephalides felis, Dipylidium, Toxocara canis, Toxascaris leonine* and *Ancylostoma caninum*.[8] Hook worm (*A. caninum*) was found in 83% (of 163) of dogs and puppies and tapeworm (*D. caninum*) was in 28% of the same animals. Ascarids were found in 64% of 36 dogs. Fleas and mange (sarcoptic) were also "very common." In the 1960s, the brown dog tick (*Rhipicephalus sanguineus*) appears to have been a problem (one which persists today), and owners were given information about it in the press.[9] Clearly, owners need to pay particular attention to the health of their pets with help from veterinarians, rather than use home remedies.

An idea of the current widespread nature of some dog diseases is obtained from the fact that most of the veterinary clinics saw dogs with three of the four selected diseases, Scabies, *Toxocariosis, Leptospirosis* and *Cutaneous larval migrans*.[10] Heart worm is such a common disease that it was not included in the study.[11] In the 1960s venereal tumours were "endemic," and although widespread in the roaming dog population, they were also found in owned dogs, probably as a result of uncontrolled mating.[12] Today, venereal tumours still remain common, particularly in the roaming dog population.[13] No case of rabies has ever been reported by any of the clinics. This is consistent with The Bahamas being a rabies-free country, despite some of its neighbours having rabies.[14] The percentages of all veterinary clinics diagnosing selected diseases in dogs in 1999 are given in Table 4.2. Every ten years or so, the island suffers from an outbreak of canine distemper.[15] Roaming dogs or dogs which are rarely taken to the veterinary are at most risk of dying from the virus; in many cases, this means potcakes.[16]

Table 4.2: Percentages of all veterinary clinics diagnosing selected diseases in dogs in 1999.

Disorder	% clinics reporting (n=5)
Scabies	100
Toxocariosis	80
Leptospirosis	80
Cutaneous larval migrans	20
Toxoplasmosis	0

Where possible, veterinarians attempt to educate owners and children on pet care and they have been responsible for educational articles in the press, even if they have sometimes dwelt on the dangers of "stray" dogs.[17] Veterinarians admit that they still need to do more to educate their customers.[18]

Activities of the Animal Control Unit

The Animal Control Unit is the designated competent authority responsible for the dog pound. It was conceived following the 1942 Act concerning dogs and it was initially run by the Bahamas Humane Society. The Animal Control Unit has been in its current form since the mid-1960s, when the Department of Agriculture assumed control of it. It is responsible, amongst other things, for catching roaming and nuisance dogs, raccoons, snakes and other animals. It enforces the Dog License Act, inspects guard-dog facilities, and assists the police with enforcement of the Penal Code and the Veterinary Division with animal quarantine. It receives unwanted animals directly from owners. Dogs which come to the Animal Control Unit are held for four days prior to being killed by euthanasia. When possible, adoptable animals coming into the Animal Control Unit are passed to the Bahamas Humane Society.

The Animal Control Unit currently[19] has a staff of nine, three vans for catching animals and a number of traps. The Unit operates between 8.00 a.m. and 4.00 p.m. Monday to Friday, and is closed at weekends and public holidays. A summary of the dogs impounded by the Animal Control Unit for the period 1990–1999 is given in Table 4.3. The estimated numbers of the total canines caught are given in Figure 4.1.[20] The average number of canines caught per year is 1,414 (s.e.: 130.1), the total number of canines caught during this 10-year period is therefore about 14,000.

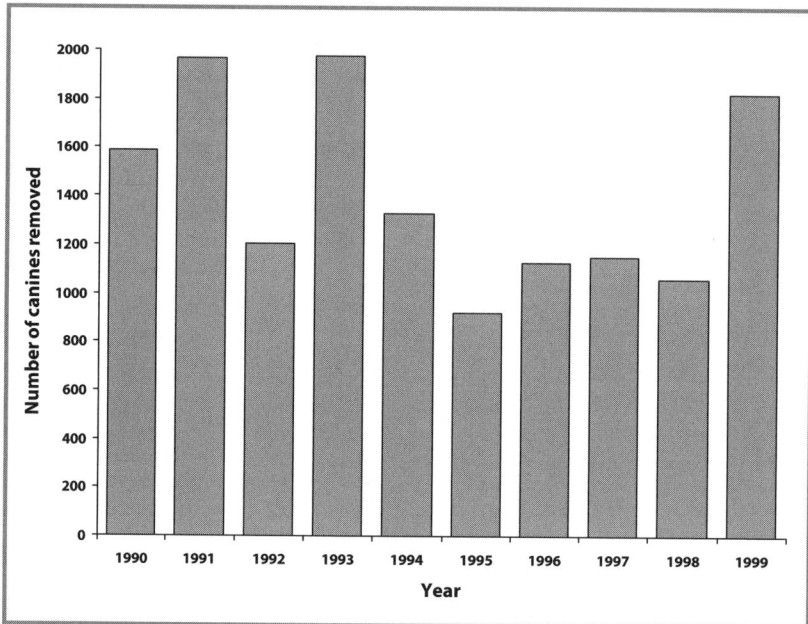

Figure 4.1: Estimated numbers of canines caught by the Animal Control Unit from 1990–1999 (figures adjusted for missing values).

Table 4.3 gives a breakdown of the overall canine catch figures. For 1990–1993, the number of dogs is probably the total number of canines, as no figures were given for the number of pups. Where very sparse data were available, no attempt has been made to provide comparative yearly figures, hence the blanks in the table.

Several consistent features are noted in Table 4.3. The percentage of dogs killed by euthanasia is close to 90% for each year. Those not killed by euthanasia were adopted, escaped or returned to their owners. An average of about 1,200 calls were made per year and about 1,250 adults removed from the dog populations, both owned and unowned; this may represent about 2% of the population. The Animal Control Unit not only offers an important service in removing unwanted or nuisance animals but its captures also help in restraining the growth of the roaming dog population.

Table 4.3: Comparative yearly figures of canines processed by the Animal Control Unit, 1990–1999.

Year	Calls made	Dogs caught	Pups caught	Dogs died (%)	Dogs adopted (%)	Dogs escaped (%)	Dogs released (%)	Dogs euthanized (%)
1990		1,586*				1	2	90
1991		1,966*		5			3	95
1992		1,204*		5		2	3	85
1993	2,144	1,974*		1		1	3	
1994		842	506		1	1	7	
1995		713	210					
1996	561	760	446	4	5	3	5	92
1997		1,152	871					
1998		1,059	938					
1999	796	1,066	794	4	3	1	6	90
Average	1,167	1,120	538	4	3	2	4	90

*For 1990–1993, the number of dogs is probably the total number of canines as no figures were given for the number of pups. As a result, the summation of the average totals for number of dogs and pups caught does not equal the average number of canines caught, 1,414. Yearly total figures have been adjusted to account for missing monthly data.

A detailed summary of the activities of the Unit for 1999 is given in Table 4.4.

Table 4.4: A summary of the numbers of animals etc. caught by the Animal Control Unit in 1999.

Dogs caught	1,066
Pups caught	784
Cats caught	52
Kittens caught	34
Raccoons caught	6
Snakes caught	2
Wild birds caught	1
Goats caught	1
Dogs returned to owner	62
Dogs adopted	33
Animals killed by euthanasia	1,678

The Unit has been criticized for being under-resourced and for failing to operate when dogs are most active,[21] namely in the early morning and evening. In recent years, the Unit has benefited from several donations of equipment and training from overseas experts and local animal rights organizations.[22] However, the contradictory attitudes of residents towards dog catching also constrain the work of the Unit. While many residents welcome the removal of roaming dogs, particularly those who do not own dogs, others threaten dog catchers, and sometimes they need police protection.[23]

The Unit is important, as it provides a legal means by which the public can get nuisance dogs removed. Thus, any inability of the Unit either to respond to calls or to catch nuisance dogs may result in residents removing these animals by whatever means they can employ.

Bahamas Kennel Club

This was founded in 1978 and is primarily a registration body that keeps records and issues certificates of pedigree to all recognized breeds of pure-bred dogs. Its registrations are accepted by kennel clubs in Canada, the UK and the USA. Its objectives include the encouragement and development of pure-bred dogs and it also strives for the better care and control of all dogs. The Club has fought against breed-specific bans, as it maintains that irresponsible dog owners, not dogs, cause "problems." Responsible dog ownership can be realized by education. To this end, the Club has organized many workshops and since 1981 it has hosted dog shows.[24] The potcake was given its own standard (see Chapter 3) in the early 1980s with the aim of bringing it respectability. There is a potcake class in all the Club's shows. The current president of the Club owns potcakes, which she has rescued herself.[25]

Animal House

Although this is a commercial grooming and boarding institution, it also provides free services directly related to animal welfare. Its staff collects dogs from the streets and, after due treatment, offers them for adoption at no cost. It will also accept unwanted animals and puts them up for adoption. It has many "non-paying guests" as boarders and a reputation of assisting dogs which might otherwise suffer. Data collected during the first three months of 2002 indicate that Animal House adopts out one animal a week; the breeds of 17 animals were recorded and of these, 16 (94%) were potcakes, and the last a poodle. All the dogs except the poodle were puppies. The sex was recorded of 19 animals; of these, 74% were females. This might suggest that owners are more inclined to abandon female than male dogs.

During the ten years it has been open, the proprietors have noticed only a single yearly peak in the numbers of puppies presented or found. They feel that pit bulls and other "dangerous" dogs have only become abundant since the mid-1990s.

Animal welfare groups

Animals Require Kindness

There are several animal welfare groups on the island. The most established of these is Animals Require Kindness, which was formed in 1991. In 1999, it had a membership of about 150. Its main thrust is a neutering programme that is free to owners. The organization raises funds for these operations, which are then carried out by the local veterinarians via a coupon system. Animals Require Kindness pays for about 780 animals a year (over 75% are on dogs, of which 75% are spays), which represents about 35% of the neuters performed at the veterinarian clinics.[26] This neutering programme is particularly successful, as the organization provides transport to get the animals to and from the clinic. Many owners cannot or will not transport their animals to the clinic, so even if they could afford the operation the animal would never receive it without the group's assistance. The importance of the transportation of pets has been observed in the neuter programme in another island.[27] It is clear that any neuter programme will have limited impact if it expects owners to bring their animals into the clinic. Funding and staffing are major constraints to the group's expanding its activities.

Advocates for Animal Rights

This group, of over 250 members, has carried out research projects associated with animal welfare, worked on revision of the legislation concerning animals and provides education to poorer animal owners. It has been an advocate of animal issues to government. It also assists animals in distress and brings cases of animal cruelty to the attention of the authorities. In recent years it has increasingly become an information source on animal issues.

Other groups

In addition to these formal groups, there are a number of individuals who help owners to better look after their animals, capture and take dogs to the clinics, and generally provide help that the larger groups, for whatever reason, fail to give.[28]

In 2001, Animal Welfare Activists Reforming Education was formed with the aim of getting pet welfare and pet care issues incorporated into the school curriculum.[29]

Co-operative initiatives

A programme involving the Rotary Club, Bahamas Humane Society, Animal Control Unit, and private veterinary clinics and utilizing corporate sponsorship started in 2002.[30] This community-based initiative targets areas which are deemed to suffer most from the problem of dog overpopulation. Rotary assists with sponsoring the neutering component, the Bahamas Humane Society and the private veterinary clinics provide the neutering services, the Animal Control Unit removes unwanted dogs and enforces the Dog Licence Act, while all participants assist with public education. Residents of the communities are actively encouraged to participate in all aspects of the programme. Each area is focused upon for one month, with follow-up, and as of September 2003, six communities had been visited.

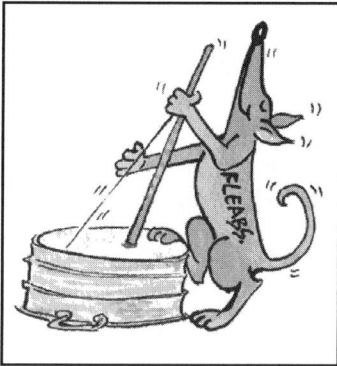

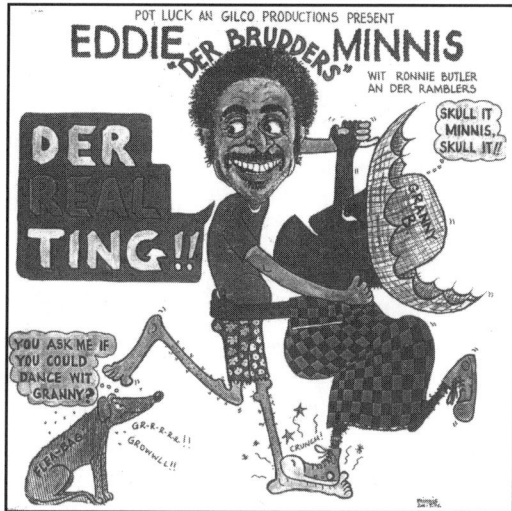

Two cartoons of potcakes in popular Bahamian culture. Fleabag clearly enjoys life but is also depicted as Granny's watchdog on an early Minnis LP record cover. (Courtesy of Eddie Minnis.)

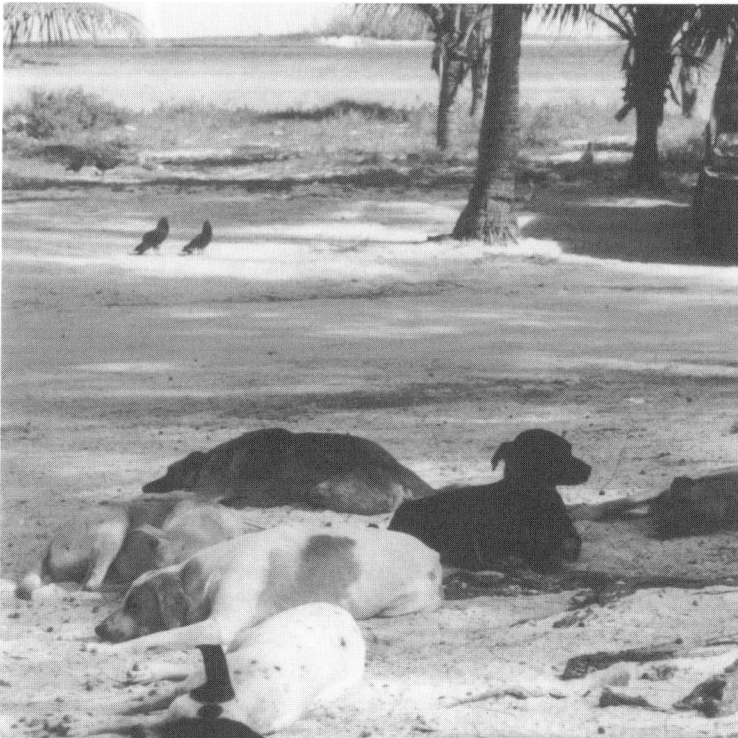

Some early commentators described New Providence's dogs as "lazy" or "aimiable." Pot-cakes are usually very docile, but they are also alert and ready for a free lunch.

This photograph of Nellie, from about 1928, is one of the first to feature a potcake. (Courtesy of the Bahamas Historical Society.)

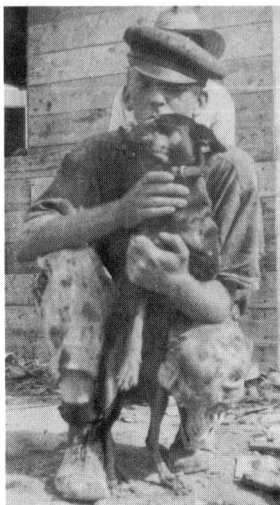

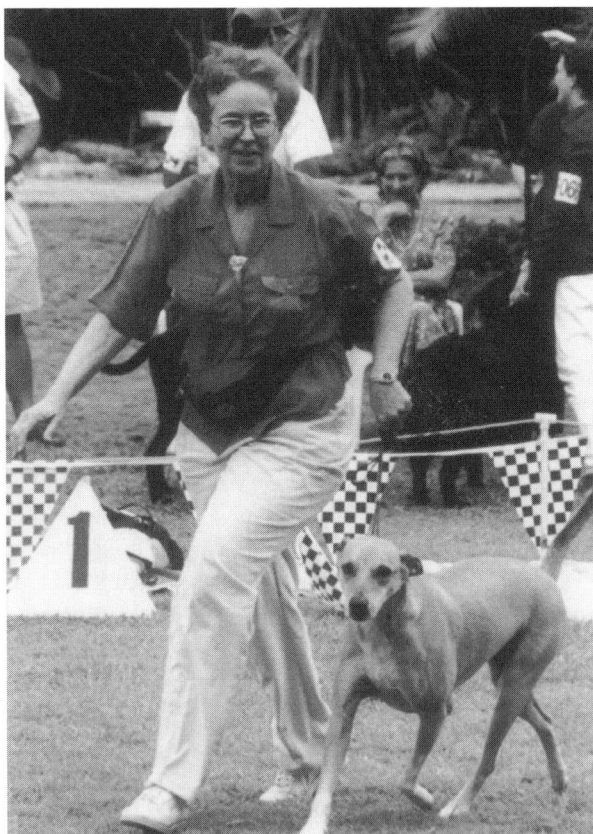

Although most Bahamians consider the potcake to be a mongrel, the Bahamas Kennel Club acknowledges the potcake as a breed. Mikhail, pictured here, was a winner of the potcake class of the Bahamas Kennel Club Dog Show and so might be considered to be a classic potcake. (Courtesy of Val Albury.)

5

What Is a "Pet"?

The majority of dogs in Nassau are mongrels which no one would want as pets . . .[1]

In The Bahamas, dogs are commonly regarded as pets, and so, depending upon one's cultural upbringing, this word can elicit expectations as to how these dogs should be kept. Therefore, we raise the issue as to what is considered to be a pet in the Bahamian context. An understanding of this concept is important, as it is easy to use foreign views to determine what a pet is and then apply those ideas in judging how "pets" are kept in The Bahamas.[2]

In order to assess what is understood by a pet in The Bahamas, first-year students in the School of Education at The College of The Bahamas were asked to identify which of 18 animals they considered to be a pet, and which of them they would own as a pet.[3] They were then asked to list characteristics they associated with a pet. They were not limited as to how many characteristics they could choose.

They were also asked to examine the importance of seven reasons why their neighbours kept dogs. We used this approach to find out reasons of ownership, because while dogs are owned by many people, dog ownership is very uneven and personal. Within a household, dogs are often considered to belong to one person,[4] and so many non-responses would have been obtained if these questions had been asked only of dog owners. Another reason for posing the question this way was that it made students assess the behaviour of their neighbours towards dogs. This prevented them answering questions on their personal ownership, which might have resulted in them giving answers that they felt might be expected or "correct." However, by answering questions about the actions of their neighbours, they effectively gave information about the actions of each other.

In addition, four focus groups, each of about nine students from the School of Education, were held which addressed the issues of "What is a pet?" and "What is responsible pet ownership?"

What is a "pet"?

One hundred and twenty trainee teachers (93% females) with a median age of 20 years (Range: 17–41) provided replies. Twenty-two percent were dog owners. Fifty-seven percent lived in households with children. All 18 animals were considered eligible to be pets, but larger animals were less likely to be chosen for a pet than smaller animals, and none actually wished to have a pig as a pet (Table 5.1). "My granddaddy, he had goats and turkey and cows—but they weren't pets, they were like a source of food." This comment, together with the responses in Table 5.1, shows that animals most often associated with farms were not generally considered as pets.

Table 5.1: A summary of the percentages of 120 Bahamian college students who considered and would own selected animals as pets.

Animal	Considered as a pet %	Would own as a pet %
Fish	98	78
Dogs	98	71
Cats	98	66
Birds	94	68
Rabbits	92	48
Hamsters	88	39
Turtles	85	47
Gerbils	50	18
Horses	44	8
Guinea pigs	40	12
Snakes	38	5
Spiders	25	4
Frogs	23	2
Goats	22	5
Chickens	20	4
Pigs	19	0
Cows	13	1
Rats	12	1

This list shows important differences in the choice of creatures as a pet compared with other societies.[5] For example, fish and rabbits seem to be particularly favoured. However, the range of animals imported as pets into The Bahamas is limited to mainly dogs, cats, fish, birds, turtles, rabbits, hamsters, guinea pigs and gerbils[6]; this list also includes the top eight animals in Table 5.1. It might be possible that the availability of creatures as pets influences what people perceive to be a pet. That is, if the creature is in a pet shop it must, by definition, be a pet. The rankings of the animals in Table 5.1 highlight the approval of fish, cats, dogs and birds as pets. These creatures were also the commonly mentioned ones in the focus groups, and so the discussion of these groups is consistent with the choice of pets indicated in Table 5.1. Although fish were favoured as a pet in our study, other studies[7] have not found this. Why Bahamians like fish so much as pets we have yet to investigate.

When children were in a household, rabbits were more likely to be considered to be a pet than when children were absent—97% vs. 86%, p=0.036). Conversely, cows were less likely to be considered a pet when children were present than when no child was in the household (8% vs. 21% respectively, p=0.051). The presence of children was not associated with any other preferences (p>0.24).

Although this study of young people found that 43% (seven replies) of males were dog owners and 23% (96 replies) of females were dog owners, the number of males was too low for the difference to be statistically confirmed. In our pet attachment study (see below), 92% (of 36) of male students lived in dog owning households, compared to 73% (of 40) of females students (p=0.04); and 19% (of 36) of male and 44% (of 41) female students (p=0.029) lived in cat owning households.[8] These observations may suggest that young men are more associated with dogs and young women more with cats, which confirms a common perception that women like dogs less than men do. The attachment study also found that in 76 households, 66% of them had dogs only, 16% had cats only and 16% had both cats and dogs. Thus, the presence of one of these pets often excludes the other (p<0.001).

The attributes associated with pets can be divided into two groups, one where the owner was the giver, and other where the pet was the giver; for example, "something to care for" and "offers loyalty." These answers show interesting differences in the role of a pet. Some of the more commonly suggested attributes associated with pets are given in Table 5.2. Attributes which were mentioned only once have been omitted for compactness of presentation. (Note that respondents were allowed to list as many attributes as they wished.) Although the ranking of items in this list follows that found elsewhere,[9] the frequency of "for love" is lower, 44% (of 27 dog owners), compared with 68% reported in America.

Neighbours primarily keep pet dogs as a protector (Table 5.3). This is again consistent with the findings of our resident perception studies, the statements from the Bahamas Kennel Club about guard dogs, and the observation that "guard dog breeds" are the type most commonly seen at veterinarian clinics. Although many owners find it convenient to use dogs as burglar alarms, such a function is not without danger to the animals. The danger to dogs as protectors was illustrated in a focus group: "and because they [five dogs] used to protect the yard so well they got bumped off . . . one got stoned and the others were poisoned." Newspapers have reported that those attempting to rob business places have killed guard dogs.[10] Dogs and security issues are discussed further in Chapter 11.

Table 5.2: A summary of attributes defining a pet by 110 Bahamian college students. (Percentages of each response by ownership class of respondent.)

Attribute	Dog owners (n=27)	Non-dog owners (n=83)
Something to love	44	33
Something to care for	37	55
Companion	33	33
Is protective	26	27
A friend	26	10
Something to treat like a child	22	2
Offers loyalty	22	11
Considered as a family member	11	14
Something kept in the home	11	7
Claimed/owned animal	11	
Animal which had been domesticated	7	3
Animal with close relationship with owner/confidant	7	1
Something to nurture		8
Something kept inside or outside the home		7
Something to be respected like a human		7
Something of owner's choice		6
Something to give attention to		6
Provides comfort		5
Source of responsibility		5
Animal which requires little effort to care for		3
For entertainment		3
Provides affection		3
Provides care		3
Something to be proud of		3
Something to bring enjoyment into the heart		3
Something to play with		3
Animal which lives with human family		2
Animal which requires attention		2
Small animal		2
Something to teach the owner responsibility		2
Something to touch		2
Source of love		2

Table 5.3: A summary of the importance for the reason as to why neighbours keep dogs as given by 120 Bahamian college students (percentages within attributes).

Attribute	Most important	Important	Slightly important	Not important
Something to make one feel safer	66	20	7	7
Companionship	28	36	21	16
Something to care for	10	36	36	18
Something to touch	4	21	34	41
A reason for exercise	4	15	39	42
A focus of attention	3	30	47	20
Something to keep one busy	3	11	39	47

While students nominated many care-related aspects as attributes of a pet, they were not perceived to be important to many of their neighbours (Table 5.3). However, when the students were divided into dog owners and non-dog owners, the responses in Table 5.3 were similar ($p > 0.10$) in both groups except for "something to touch." For that attribute, 44% of students in dog owning households thought that this was important (or more) compared with 21% of those in non-dog owning households ($p = 0.036$). This may suggest that companionship aspects, at least in a predominantly female group of respondents, may be more important than non-owners imagine.

Comments

Characteristics of what defines a creature as a "pet" were varied. A summary of these characteristics was given in Table 5.2 above. Interestingly, only 11% of dog owners considered ownership as a characteristic of a pet, and none of the non-pet owners explicitly stated that an animal had to be owned to be a pet. Ownership may have been considered to be such an obvious aspect that it was assumed.[11] An alternative explanation, that people think an animal can be a pet (or "individual") without being property,[12] particularly given the other characteristics listed, is, we feel, unlikely.

Respondents were classified as to whether or not they owned dogs. Non-dog owners appear to stress the "family member" aspect more than owners. This might be because non-owners are considering the attributes in a less practical way than owners. For example, one may like to offer the dog a place in the household, but limitations of space, the presence of small children, health issues and conflicts within the family may prevent the pet from being incorporated into the home. While 69% of owners, in our neuter study, considered dogs in human terms, only 11% of the owners in this study considered a pet as a family member and something to keep in the home. This could lead to the idea that dogs are "displaced humans." As The Bahamas becomes more "developed" (i.e., has greater resources), owners may be more able to look after their pets as they would like.

In Table 5.2 it can be seen that similar numbers of non-owners identified love, companionable and protective characters as attributes of pets. This contrasts with other studies that found love and companionability to dominate over protective aspects.[13] Perceptions of pets as companionable animals are important, as they should encourage better care and companionable pets have beneficial effects on the owners.[14] The term "companionable animal" is considered more "dignified and evocative" and suggests an animal worth more than its monetary value.[15]

The results in Table 5.2 are in broad agreement with those reported in Table 5.3, but protective aspects are clearer in Table 5.3. Thus, no matter how much owners say they love their pets (and we feel that Bahamians are probably more attached to their pets than people elsewhere[16]), in the eyes of their neighbours, they do not always turn this love of pets into action. There would appear to be barriers (which include knowledge of appropriate pet care) that prevent owners from translating their inherent attachment to animals into pet care visible to their neighbours. In Chapter 13 we pursue explanations of this further.

The areas listed in Table 5.2 are also reflected in the focus groups' discussions, where the size of the animal was mentioned as being important—"a pet would have to be something small," but also something of which the owner is "not afraid." This reasoning may explain the popularity of fish and the choice of toy breed dogs for pets (see Table 10.1 on the types of dogs imported). It may also suggest why women claimed to be less fond of pets in general than men.[17] There was a general consensus that a pet was an "animal of choice" which one cared for. However, it was agreed that no one would want a rat as a pet, but this agreement may reflect the fact that our sample was dominated by females.

Elsewhere, the choice of animal for a pet is associated with traits of the owner.[18] Our study is unable to compare the responses of males and females, but elsewhere female dog owners have been found to be more "dominant" and having more "masculine attributes" than male owners. These observations may also apply to Bahamians, where men might be insecure of their position[19] and women often run households.[20] Such gender differences may also account for differences in actions and attitudes towards the neutering of male dogs noted in our neuter study (see Chapter 12).

6

Pet Attachment

Bahamians are one of the kindest and most loving peoples on the face of the earth.[1]

It is important to assess the level of attachment which owners have, or think that they would have, to their "pets" so that their responses in surveys can be better interpreted. If people are not well attached to their pets, it might be reasonable for pets to be kept in ways that give cause for concern. However, if owners are attached to their pets but offer them little care, this may highlight issues beyond the control of owners which prevent them from looking after pets the way they wish.

The study

To assess attachment to pets, a self-assessment form, based upon an already existent one,[2] was devised consisting of 19 statements that could be answered using a scale of 1 (strongly disagree) to 7 (strongly agree) and is reproduced in the Appendix 1. Self-assessment forms of this nature have obvious limitations, but they do provide information on what people perceive their attachment to be. Users of the library at The College of The Bahamas and non-academic staff members completed this form. Respondents were categorized by gender, age and type of pets owned, if any.

The statements were phrased so that non-pet owners could still indicate their thoughts on the issues. The changes made to the original attachment statements were designed to make them more appropriate to The Bahamas; the maximum score on this form was 133.

In presenting the results from this investigation we also include relevant information from our focus groups and neuter study.

Results

As usual with self-completion forms, not all the forms were completed, so the number of valid responses was sometimes less than 165, the number of study respondents. When statements were left unanswered, it was assumed that the person was "unsure," and this default was inserted.

The respondents were 47% male and the median age was 21 years, with a minimum age of 16 years and a maximum of 59. Fifty-five percent of respondents (146 replies) had pets of some type in their household.

A score of 76 (or 57%) would indicate "not sure" to all statements and 95 (or 71%) "slightly agree" to all statements. People in pet owning households had a higher attachment to pets (97.8, se=2.39) than those in non-pet owning households (81.8, se=2.63) (p<0.001). Given the total score of 133, individuals in pet owning households had an average attachment of 74% compared to 62% for those in non-pet owning households. Thus, the overall level of attachment of respondents in pet owning households is equivalent to "slight" agreement with the statements covered. The minimum attachment level was 28 (21%) and the highest 132 (99%). The level of attachment was not influenced by gender or the presence of pets in the household (p>0.05). The levels of attachments are summarized in Table 6.1.

When responses were divided into those who disagreed and those who agreed with the statements, a number of differences were identified between individuals from pet owning and non-pet owning households, Table 6.2.[3] These responses might help to explain why people do or do not choose to be a pet owner.

Table 6.1: Summary of pet attachment, or anticipated attachment, percentage in each household type.

Average response to all questions	Pets in household (n=77)	No pets in household (n=61)	All (n=155)
More than moderately agreeing	23.4	3.3	13.5
Moderately agreeing	37.6	21.3	30.0
Agreeing somewhat	26.0	44.3	32.9
Unsure	6.5	18.0	14.9
Disagreeing somewhat	5.2	6.5	5.1
Disagreeing moderately or less	1.3	6.6	3.9

Responses from 155 individuals at The College of The Bahamas. Agreement is associated with closer attachment to pets.(Percentages in each class are those which exceed the cut-off point of the group below, up to, and including the cut-off point of the group category.)

Table 6.2: Percentages of College of The Bahamas respondents agreeing with statements concerning pet care.

Statement	Pet owning household	Non-pet owning household	P=
Pets are not a waste of money*	98	87	0.019
I like animals around the home	87	71	0.032
I like house pets	76	58	0.036
I communicate with pets	74	49	0.006
I like pets inside my home	71	45	0.003
It is better to care for pets than people	25	43	0.027

n≈75, for owning and n≈55 for non-owning pet households. The complete list of statements is given in Appendix 1.
*The reverse statement was used in the study.

Other indicators of attachment in which there were no differences (p>0.06) between individuals from pet and non-pet owning households are given in Table 6.3.

Although most respondents agreed that pets should have a place in the home (Table 6.3), in reality most dogs are kept outside and many are even allowed to roam.[4] Older respondents (over the median age of 21 years) were more likely to agree that pets should be kept outside (47% of 64 replies) than younger respondents (those under 21 or younger) (24% of 82 replies).

Female respondents appeared to be more emotionally attached to pets than males, as 73% (of 78) of females thought that they would cry when their pet died compared with 56% (of 68) of males (p=0.037). However, men seem to have a closer physical attachment to pets than women, as 53% of men (of 66) compared with 33% (of 77) of women liked to feed animals from their hands (p=0.017); yet men (51% of 67) were less willing to have pets in the home than women (68% of 78) (p=0.042).

Table 6.3: Indicators of pet attachment, or anticipated attachment, of respondents at The College of The Bahamas.

Statement	% of individuals agreeing (n≈130)
I love pets	85
I like seeing pets enjoy food	83
House pets bring happiness into my life	81
You should respect pets like human beings	73
I talk to my pet	72
I spend time playing with my pet	66
I cry when my pet dies	66
Pets damage furniture	52
I like to feed pets from my hand	42
Pets mean more to me than friends	35
Pets should be kept outside	33
Pets are fun but not worth the trouble	16
Animals belong in the wild or zoo, not in the home	12

The complete list of statements is given in Appendix 1.

The fact that only one statement ("Pets are not a waste of money") received 90% or more agreement/disagreement of respondents in both pet owning and non-owning households shows that within these groups there are conflicting opinions concerning pets. (See also the views expressed in the case studies in Chapter 7.) Conflict within a pet owning household has also been observed when interviewing residents[5]: "We only have dogs because of my husband, I would not have them otherwise"; or again: "I am not sure why we have them."

While some owners do have close relationships with their pets, it is clear that some in the focus groups thought that there were limits to acceptable dog care:

> The dogs . . . used to stay inside and afterwards became a nuisance . . . they have to stay outside. . . . They were spoilt. . . . They had a doghouse but . . . my little sister . . . they used to sleep in the bed with her. . . . They too big to stay inside . . . they still come inside and sit on the sofa and the bed sometimes.

And

> Harry [the dog's name] was cute and cuddly. Harry would sleep inside. . . . He was a chow-chow. He was different. . . . He wasn't a normal dog.

Differences between the levels of care offered to potcakes and "nice" dogs have been noted in several of our studies and were also present in the focus groups:

> What we don't want, we give it to the dog [which is kept outside].
>
> Does the animal go to the vet?
> —No . . . we are talking about potcakes here.
> So why a potcake cannot go to the vet?
>
> I mean, I [take it] personally? Because it is not my pet, I don't think I should take the responsibility of someone else's animal . . . he's a potcake—that's money.

Dogs in households with few occupants can be expected to play a more important companionable role than in larger households[6] and in industrialized countries the companionable aspects of pets are considered important.[7] In the West Indies, families are large (the modal household size was five in our neuter study), relatively few people live alone, and relations take care of the elderly.[8] Another study indicated that in smaller households—one or two people—companionable aspects of ownership could be of less importance.[9] That study suggested that as fewer than expected smaller households did not have a dog, the companionable aspects of dog ownership might not be important, possibly because of the extended family structure. However, as households fragment (the percentage of smaller households was 34% in 1990[10] and 39% in 2000[11]), companionable aspects of pet ownership may grow.

Confining dogs also increases the opportunity for bonding between owners and animals and enhances animal welfare. In the neuter study (see Chapter 12), the type of the owner's dwelling (house or apartment) did not influence whether or not dogs could roam (p=0.87). However, in households with one or two people, 32% (of 62) of owners let their dogs roam compared with 45% (of 216) of owners in larger households (p=0.08). This provides an indicator that companionable aspects may be more fully exploited in smaller households.

Comments

This exercise was undertaken to find the Bahamian context in which owners or potential owners are attached to their pets. This understanding is useful when we consider the results in our surveys so that they can be interpreted in the appropriate context.

Attachment is an important concept when discussing pets, as this is linked with the care we offer animals considered as pets. The higher the level of attachment or bonding between owner and pet, the higher the level of welfare we can expect the pet to receive. Our findings suggest that attachment between pets and those in an owning household could be greater, and understandably people in non-pet owning households are less attached to pets than those in closer contact with them. In particular, the focus groups highlighted that people may be less attached to potcakes than other types of dog, that there are limits to what people might regard as an acceptable level of attachment, and that these vary according to the type of dog. It seems that different limits apply to the attachment of pure-bred dogs compared to potcakes.

In this study 85% of the participants agreed (to various degrees) that they loved pets (Table 6.3), a figure which is in close agreement with the 83% who said that they liked "pets in general" in our perception study in New Providence. Thus both studies give a clear message that Bahamians see themselves as fond of pets. Students in pet owning households were in "slight agreement"[12] (74%; 95% confidence limits 70%–77%, compared with 71% for "slight agreement") with the issues raised in the survey. In similar studies on pet attachment owners have scored 68%[13] (on a five-point scale, 60% would indicate neutral feelings) and 67%[14] (also on a five-point scale). Although results from different scales cannot be directly compared, it would seem that Bahamians may be more attached to their pets than owners elsewhere.[15]

As one might expect, people living in non-owning households show lower levels of attachment (to abstract pets) than those living with pets. The reactions of non-owners to pets are important, as a large number of households do not own pets. However, these people, like owners, interact with roaming dogs and so can influence their welfare.

Although some gender differences were observed, other studies have found that male owners are less attached to their pets than women.[16] Those differences seen here conform to our general impressions gathered during the course of these studies. While women are less associated with pets, they are more emotionally attached to them than men. In the case of The Bahamas, while men are more associated with dogs than women, men also avail themselves of the economic opportunities which can accrue by dog breeding, in particular "image" dogs (see Chapters 10 and 12).

The fact that 32% of owners in smaller households—one or two people—still let their dogs roam suggests that owners may not fully exploit the companionable aspect of dog ownership.[17] This level of companionship between owners and pets was also seen in our study of student teachers at The College of The Bahamas, in which only 28% of them considered companionship to be a "most important" reason for neighbours' keeping dogs. However, as the family structure changes in The Bahamas, the importance of companionable aspects of pet ownership might be expected to increase.[18]

Elderly owners can be closely attached to their potcakes. An article about an old, single woman in a poorer part of Nassau provides an interesting case study and confirms our observations above. It reported that her potcakes are "constant companions . . . who are deadly serious when they bark" even if the dogs "are probably not as well-fed as the wondering mongrels of the area" and that "she will probably have a merry Christmas and stay in that house with her two dogs [potcakes] until the day she dies."[19] This is a clear example of pet companionship. One also gets the impression that she looks after the dogs as much as her material circumstances permit. Thus, despite close attachment, the level of welfare she can offer her companions might give cause for concern. This newspaper story suggests that "Granny and Fleabags" may be rooted in reality.

The results from the attachment study provide an interesting contrast to the observations that students made about why their neighbours keep dogs (Table 5.3). From the outsider's view, it is clear that dog ownership is a means of residents protecting their home, and companionable aspects are of less importance. From the personal viewpoint, love and companionable aspects are foremost. These conflicting views could be reconciled through the suggestion that owners, while loving their pets, fail to translate their concept of love into clear actions. One reason for this could be that 33% of those in the study (Table 6.3) thought that dogs should be kept outside, and this group gives the impression to outsiders that all owners keep their dogs (outside) for protection. It should be noted that Bahamians are not alone in having positive feelings towards their pets, but are unable to "translate these feelings into more animal friendly practices,"[20] as similar observations have been made in Costa Rica.[21]

Alternatively, there may be economic pressures that prevent pet loving owners from converting their affection for their pets into actions. Comments from a focus group show a reluctance to spend money on a potcake. This reluctance could be due to economic constraints or a simple perception that one does not spend money on potcakes. However, if money were not an issue, we feel that owners would be willing to offer more care to potcakes and pets, as even 87% of those in non-owning households thought that pets were not a waste of money (Table 6.2). Some economic considerations are discussed in Chapter 13 and they also surface in the case studies described in Chapter 7.

A report of an owner who saved his car from a fire rather than prevent his rottweiler from being burnt is a graphic example of an owner being forced to put his attachment to his dog to the test.[22] Here was a valuable dog, kept inside the house, whose barking saved his owner's life, but the owner appears to have chosen to let the animal perish rather than allow his even more valuable car to be destroyed. While this example might seem to show limits to attachment (as noted in the focus groups), it is an extreme example of how owners sometimes have to make harsh economic decisions concerning their resources. This event contrasts with a publicized memorial service for "Taco Strachan," a two-year-old Chihuahua, a pet that was clearly loved by its owners,[23] who live in a poorer inner-city area. The depth of pet attachment which some owners have was described in a letter to the press[24] which stressed the psychological damage caused in dog loving households when pets are stolen.

Overall, our findings could be taken to mirror the picture painted by Minnis of Granny's attachment to Fleabag. Granny loves her faithful, barking potcake Fleabag. However, barriers are (probably) present which prevent her from providing him with health care. To an outsider, Granny could be seen to keep Fleabags for protection and not to really care for him because of his fleas (or poor health).

7

Responsibilities of Owners Towards Pets

> And a public education campaign focusing on the re-
> sponsibilities involved in animal ownership, not just
> dogs, should be conducted.[1]

"Responsible pet ownership" has been much discussed in the media and it is deemed
essential if the roaming dog problem is to be solved.[2] However, in the absence of formal
education on pet welfare this is a vague concept which seems to be little understood.
Various groups have offered definitions as to what "responsible pet ownership" means;
for example:

> Animal ownership carries with it a dual responsibility: The animal owner has a re-
> sponsibility to his neighbour to ensure that his animal does not commit any tres-
> pass against his neighbour, and the animal owner has a responsibility to the animal
> for its care and wellbeing.[3]

Even if such a definition lacks detail, it is clear that animal ownership can be onerous if
a high level of care is to be given the pet. Legally, owners have few defined responsibilities that they must execute on behalf of their pets (for example, they are not obliged to
offer any regular health care), but certain actions relating to animal cruelty are pro-
scribed under the Penal Code.[4] These relate to intentional cruelty, starvation, tethering
"without a proper supply of food or water" and "mistreatment."

According to law, owners are not allowed to urge "any dog or other animal to attack, worry or put in fear any person or animal." If a dog causes an injury, a previous
"mischievous propensity in the dog" must be shown or "neglect on the part of the
owner" before any compensation can be claimed.[5] Thus, while society does not place
extraordinary expectations on dog owners, they are required to control their animal,
particularly if it is "large . . . ferocious dog," and be responsible for its actions. Official

advice goes further and asks that owners neuter, confine, and provide health care for their dogs, and not feed dogs that they do not own.[6]

In order to find out what Bahamians understand responsible pet ownership to be, we report the findings of some focus groups and case studies.[7] Such information allows interpretation of "responsible pet ownership" in a Bahamian context, and lets us find out how people think pets, and dogs in particular, should be treated.

The focus group participants, students in Education at The College of The Bahamas,[8] agreed that "good pet ownership is treating the animal the way you want to be treated . . . shelter . . . food . . . water . . . affection . . . health care, exercise" and neutering. These responsibilities are also found in the list of attributes associated with pets listed in Chapter 6.

There was also general agreement that their neighbours did not look after their pets, with comments such as:

> they have no regard for dogs
>
> my neighbours do not care about their animals at all . . . their ribs are sticking out
>
> the dogs have fleas dripping off them. It looks like water just dripping . . . and the food that they give them is bad . . .

There were general complaints about dogs being allowed to roam and how this resulted in garbage bins being knocked over and making the streets unsafe: "they have really bad dogs like pit bulls and sometimes they get into the street."

However, the characteristics of responsible pet ownership, while reflecting those in the media, were not always seen in the way in which group members actually looked after their own pets:

> we would give them [dogs] the left-over food. The bone, the chicken . . . whatever we didn't eat. Sometimes I would bathe them but they usually get their shower when it rained. They lived on the outside.

These contradictory statements are consistent with the observations made in Chapter 6, and result in the pets receiving limited care. Although people may be able to say how others should look after their pets, they seem unable to follow their own advice.

The reactions from the focus groups with students towards responsible pet ownership were similar to those obtained from two in-depth case study interviews.

Two case studies

These detailed interviews provided an opportunity to understand the actions and perceptions of two owners towards dog ownership. Further, their answers could often be verified through direct observation. The ability to check what the interviewees said with their actions is important in differentiating between what people say they do or think that they do and what they actually do. Hence, the information from these interviews might also suggest alternative interpretations or qualifications to inferences made in our other studies.

Case study 1[9]

Miss F. was 30 years old and lived in the southeastern area of central Nassau; she owned six dogs.

Miss F. was an unmarried cashier who lived with five other family members from four generations in a three-bedroom bungalow. There was a small front yard and a larger, but still small, back yard. The front yard faced the road and was not fenced. The back yard primarily consisted of bare earth, contained much rubbish and adjoined an area of bush. The back yard fence was dilapidated and not stock-proof. The grandfather complained that the back yard was too small for so many dogs and that the yard was "unsanitary," despite the faeces being cleaned up by Miss F. Her mother, who washed the dogs once a month,[10] complained that the dogs liked to "wallow in the dirt."

Her family has a history of owning dogs, as her parents and grandparents had dogs. She learnt how to care for her dogs from her family; she was taught nothing at school about pet care. The only book she had on pet care was about rabbits. All their dogs, and hers, were obtained from friends (but see inconsistency below).

Sometimes her mother brought home a dog she saw on the street, and this was why they had so many dogs. These dogs were a female, seven-year-old Chihuahua; a four-year-old, female Labrador mixed with rottweiler; a female, eight-year-old retriever mix; two potcakes, both three years old, one male and one female; and a male potcake of unknown age. One male and one female were "fixed"; the operations were paid for by her mother and done at the Bahamas Humane Society. All nine pups of one litter died. Three pups of another litter (original size unknown) were still alive; all these pups had been reserved by friends. Only one litter was planned from a selected dog (but all the pups—five, she thinks—died). She thought her male dog was responsible for all the other "accidents."

She fed the dogs on tinned pet food each day together with six "scoops" of dried dog food. She sometimes mixed in household scraps, such as rice mixed with vegetables and meat (chicken, including the bones), so that they got a "balanced meal." However, she conceded that "you should not really feed them table scraps." She did not feed them fish bones. Her dogs also ate fruits, such as apples and bananas.[11] The dried dog food was kept in a cooler and she bought canned dog meat by the case from a wholesale supermarket. When the usual brands were unavailable she changed the diet accordingly.

She did not exercise the dogs, but the "house dog" was taken out sometimes.

She, like the parents and grandparents, owned dogs because she "loves" them. Miss F. "loves animals" and her love of animals extended beyond dogs, as she had had many different pets while growing up. She considered dogs more as "part of the family" than as pets, and people should "look after animals like children." The protection that dogs could offer a household was not a consideration in keeping them, although that aspect was acknowledged. Her dogs "bark a lot" and in 26 years, their home had never been broken into. She considered a pet to be a "gentle" and "obedient" animal which could be "taken into the home." Only her Chihuahua came inside the house (the house dog), as it was a small dog.[12] There was not enough room inside for the family and the larger dogs. Her sister was worried that the children "may pick-up something" from the dogs.[13] Her grandparents kept their dogs outside, but her mother "would sleep with them." The rottweiler mix was kept in the front yard and the others in the back yard. The reason for this dog being kept in the front yard was because he "jumps the fence." Sometimes she had to chain the dogs to stop them fighting, but they always had access to shade and water.

Although one of her dogs can roam, she thought that "He only goes to the neighbour and back." She did not think that "stray" dogs could get inside the yard, even though one of her dogs could jump out over the fence. The roaming dogs in the neighbourhood were "infested with fleas and ticks" and they had undermined her efforts to keep her dogs free from these disorders:"[I] cannot take care of my dogs because of strays." She realized that keeping her dogs outside did not help their health.

She considered her dogs to be "healthy" except for some "skin problems." All the animals except the pups had had their "shots." She has planned to get the other animals "fixed" when they were no longer in heat and she had no objection to neutering males. She had never caught a disease from a dog. She would take the animals to the vet "when needed," and considered "vets . . . expensive, but [they are] worth it." She had sprayed the garden once to get rid of ticks.

One of her previous dogs had been killed on the road and another one, which had its back broken by a car, was put to sleep.

A friend licensed three of her dogs but she did not know how to get the licenses herself. She had the dogs licensed so that they could be returned to her should they get lost.

In her opinion, a "responsible" pet owner must make sure the dog got its "shots" (vaccinations), went to the veterinarian, was fed, loved and exercised. She thinks that more people were responsible pet owners than before. It was wrong to let a dog roam, as "anything can happen to it."

"Stray" dogs had bred behind her house (in the bush) and were fed by people in the neighbourhood. The previous residents had moved away and apparently left the dogs behind. She did not intentionally feed animals, but "stray" dogs did eat the food that she puts out for her dogs. Birds also came and ate the food that the dogs left. Garbage was stored in an enclosure with a top, so "the dogs can't get at it." She had no suggestion as what could be done about the unwanted dogs and felt that she could do nothing herself to alleviate the problem.

She viewed the "stray" dog problem as the owners' fault. Dogs should be "fixed." She saw no evidence of the government dog-catchers (Animal Control Unit). She felt that the roaming dog "problem" was "getting worse" and she was "seeing more dogs."

Miss F. felt there were too many uncared for dogs and irresponsible owners should be fined.

Miss F. said that people who do not look after their dogs properly did not want to be told what to do. She thought that people needed more education about pet care. Seminars, open to all, should be given and information should be provided in all the media. Humane societies should do more and the public should give them more support. The public should have access to free neuter programmes.

Dog ownership has taught her responsibility and how to interact with people. She considered herself to be an "excellent pet owner" and as a "responsible" pet owner.

Interviewer's observations

Miss F. has been helped in the past by an animal welfare group to have some animals neutered and treated by the veterinarian for injuries. She has not had any further animals neutered herself. The health of all her animals was poor. Miss F. did not know that her dogs had allergies or what to do with them. The Chihuahua (which was allowed inside the house with the children) was clearly sick. This dog received considerable human contact, as it sat on Miss F.'s lap during the interview. One dog had runny eyes, and two were pregnant or had pups. All the animals had skin disorders. Although the dogs could not be aged, the ages given for all the dogs seemed exaggerated; none of the dogs looked old. The yard was not an appropriate place to keep the animals. It was clear that roaming dogs could get in, and probably her dogs could also get out. The dog in the front yard could easily roam, and old wounds from fights were visible.

Case study 2

Mr. M., who was about 35 years old and owned two dogs, went to high school, and now worked in the family business while he was studying to get his realtor's license; previously, he was a reserve policeman. He lived with his parents and four siblings in a four-bedroom house on the eastern edge of Nassau. His daughter, together with numerous nephews and nieces (aged between 2–10 years old) were daily visitors to the house.

Until very recently, Mr. M. owned three dogs, but one died so he now had a rottweiler and a rottweiler–German shepherd mix (one male and one female). Both pets were nine years old and unlicensed. One was acquired, in poor condition, from its previous owner, who bred guard dogs. His previous dogs (potcakes) were obtained through adoption, as gifts, some were "found" and others bought. Formerly, he allowed his dogs to roam, but the current ones did not.

He has "always" had dogs, usually potcakes, and his father had dogs, although he was also fond of cats. He regarded his family as a "family of animal lovers," although his sisters, who were not tall, preferred smaller dogs to the larger ones he had. His grandparents had a dog, which was killed by a car when the dog got onto the road. Mr. M. learnt much about pet care from his parents, in particular, the importance of taking the pet to the veterinarian when it was sick. He also learnt more from veterinarians and later he bought books on dog care.

Mr. M.'s dogs lived in a fenced-in yard and they also had access to a large shed and a "full sized" dollhouse, but they preferred to use the shed. He took the dogs for walks, played with them in the yard, and took them for drives and on visits to the beach. They rarely went inside the house. His father helped with the care of the dogs.

Mr. M. kept dogs because he "loves animals." He regarded a pet as a "friend that has no limits, no boundaries . . . and it will love you back." He noted that the dogs had become protective of him without any training—they seemed to protect "by instinct." He also pointed out that his dogs distinguished between adults and children, and while they may bark at the former, they did not bark at the latter, and they were tolerant of the way children handle them. He felt that "a good pet owner" was one who was "willing to treat animals as they treat themselves."

Mr. M.'s pets rarely came inside the house because of the children. His sisters were wary of such big dogs around the toddlers, and they were scared of the dogs. However, he believed that children should be reared with dogs so as to foster the human-animal bond from an early age.

His female dog was spayed after its first heat and had had no pups. The male mated with a (now deceased) female and 11 of the 12 pups survived. Another female had had one litter of 13 (two of which died), and they had to be fed by hand, which was tiring and expensive, but pups had to be treated "like babies." A few pups were sold, but the remainder were given away to "good homes." Finding a good home was more important than making money from the pups.

Both animals had had their "shots" and probably visited the veterinarian at least once a year. One dog had a skin problem, but this had been resolved by a change of diet (suggested by the veterinarian) and medicine. When dogs were sick they were quickly taken to the clinic ("I have no hesitation in calling the emergency number of the [Bahamas] Humane Society at weekends"). When the dog became old he tried to let it pass on "naturally," but if it was very sick and in obvious pain, then he would have it put down. Use of euthanasia was a "difficult decision," but he would never want to see an animal suffer.

Typically, the dogs were fed dried food; however, as "special treats" they were given "selected" table scraps, such as "chicken meat" or "slices of cooked ham" or "larger bones."

Mr. M. considered that to be a responsible pet owner one had to "do the same for the pet as for yourself. . . . Watch them, [give them things to] eat, drink." He considered dogs to be smarter than children. Pet owners should look after their pets with "great care, love and affection."

Mr. M. perceived there to be a "stray dog problem" that was caused by people who were "negligent pet owners." Such people often "do not even look after themselves"; they allowed their pets to roam and did not take care of them. He saw the "biggest fault" of pet ownership to be that "nobody bothers to restrain their dogs." The lack of stock-proof fences and identification tags made it difficult to find owners of roaming dogs, and so to fine people for acts of cruelty. Mr. M. would not suggest how he would go about "solving" the "stray dog problem" if he had to. He seemed to think that the government should be responsible for addressing the problem, and that a "full-time organization" should deal with the issue. He suggested that many of the free-roaming dogs would have to be put down. Neuter programmes would be useful. He was of the opinion that the government "does not consider it a problem which requires immediate attention." However, he indicated that the government's animal control officers should be more vigilant and more active in catching animals.

Mr. M. suggested that the number of dogs a household has depended upon the size of the yard. No more than two dogs should be kept in a 21.3m × 27.4m yard. He thought that the current fines associated with animal cruelty were a "joke" and that people must be made aware of the repercussions of their actions: "People on the street work on the basis, 'if I do this, this will happen'. . . . Socially it is acceptable to abandon an animal. . . . Acceptance of these actions is a result of low finances, poor education and peer pressure."

Mr. M. considered pet ownership to be a "privilege," and that the owner gained more from the arrangement than the pet.

Interviewer's comments

The dogs looked healthy with good coats and clear eyes, despite their age. The yard was clean; the dogs had the use of a large doghouse as well as something rather like a child's dollhouse. The fence was stock-proof. The dogs were fed two cups of dried dog food and one can of dog food once a day.

Comments

Miss F.

Miss F. reiterates many points made in the focus groups and which are apparent in the perception studies on good pet care, while not seeing the deficiencies in the care she gives her dogs. She fails her own definition of a "responsible pet owner," yet thinks of herself as an "excellent" pet owner. It is unlikely that most pet owners would view themselves as anything less, as each owner would probably automatically view his/her standard of pet care as being the "right" one.

Few would dispute her definition of a "responsible" pet owner, namely that such a person should ensure the dog:

- gets its shots,
- goes to the vet,
- is fed,
- is loved,
- is exercised, and
- is not allowed to roam.

However, it is interesting to note that the legal requirement to license the animal was not seen as a duty of the "responsible" owner. This suggests that licensing the dog is not deemed important, a view that goes back to Powles in 1888. When these criteria are considered together with her definition of a pet as an animal which:

- is gentle
- is obedient
- can be "taken into the home,"

then only Miss F.'s Chihuahua is a "pet," as the other dogs cannot come into the home.

She has probably inherited her standards of pet care from her family, and while she may look after her pets more than her forebears, her knowledge of animal health is insufficient to know when the dogs need to see a vet. It is interesting that she did not know the number of pups born in a recent litter. This suggests that she takes only minimal interest in the dogs kept outside. It will be noted that it was her mother who was washing the dogs and the grandfather who complained about the mess in the yard due to there being too many dogs in a small space. There seems to be a feeling that the dogs are owned at two levels; (1) specific dogs belong to a particular person, (2) other dogs belong to both her and her mother, as "she" has dogs which her mother brought in off the road. Miss F. feeds the dogs but her mother carries out other tasks associated with the dogs' well-being.

While she knows what she should do for her pets, she fails to provide the desired level of care; this is illustrated by her failure to confine her dogs and the fact that she feeds table scraps[14] when she knows she should not do so. Although she thinks that her back yard is stock-proof, it clearly is not. (Many people in the resident perception studies claimed that their yards were stock-proof, but this example suggests that the reported perception may be faulty and that many more owned dogs might have access to the streets than admitted by owners.) She has a perfectly rational explanation as to why she allows one of her dogs to roam, and defends the dog's roaming by her perception that the dog does not roam far. She has no idea what the dog may do on these unsupervised walks, and she does not see her action towards this dog as "wrong"; this view may be shared by other owners who let their dogs roam.[15]

Miss F. displays a resignation about the "stray dog problem" but does not see the way she keeps her pets as contributing to the "problem." Firstly, her dogs can roam, even if she does not "allow" them to roam. The fact that two of her three females were unintentionally bred is a probable consequence of this. Further, while she knows that roaming dogs steal the food she puts out for own dogs, she has not revised her feeding methods to prevent this. This suggests that she does not feel sufficiently strongly on this issue to change her behaviour. The reason for this is probably that she, like 93% of the residents of New Providence, feels sorry for roaming dogs.[16] The habit of owners to feed dogs outside might have contributed to the apparent increase in the populations of rock doves (*Columba livia*), also called pigeons, and ring necked doves or Eurasian collared doves (*Streptopelia decaocto*).[17] In addition to benefiting from food left for dogs, the birds can be a health hazard to both the dogs and the public.

Although she does not suggest that her knowledge of pet care is deficient, she advocates the need for lessons in pet care for grown-ups. While it is clear to her that other people do not know how to look after their dogs (with the implication that she does) she makes the point that these people do not wish to learn. Presumably, such people would not attend pet care classes. It suggests that either they, like her, are satisfied with their knowledge of pet care, or giving additional care to their pets is not important to them; such people would probably not attend the seminars. The suggestion for pet care classes probably reflects her view that other people need them. Attitudes such as these are observed in other aspects of human behaviour. They also make it harder to encourage adults to change their pet care practices and so reinforce the need to teach pet care to children and to get them to influence their parents.

Like other owners, she regards her dogs "like children," an observation which stands scientific scrutiny.[18] However, she sees nothing wrong in these "children" being outside in a poorly kept yard. The household's children have priority for the limited space inside, and so despite her description, the dogs do have a lower level of care than children.

Life expectancy and infant mortality are common indicators of health and well-being. Given the lack of health care, we find it hard to accept the ages given by Miss F. for her dogs; all the ages exceed the average of three years found in our other studies. As she has no reason to know their ages, unreliable information is to be expected. The fact that only three pups have survived from two litters is an indicator of the health of her dogs.

She attributes the reason for the home not having been broken into to the presence of the dogs. However, studies have shown that criminals tend to avoid homes which are usually occupied[19] and homes in which the same people have been living for many years; thus the effectiveness of the dogs maybe a misattribution.[20] From reports on crime in the press, it is clear that even three dogs (a potcake and two Labradors) in and around the house need not deter the determined criminal.[21]

Mr. M.

An obvious result of Mr. M.'s level of health care is that he has old dogs which can still enjoy life, and whose company Mr. M. can enjoy. The presence of an effective stock-proof fence helps these dogs to maintain their health; although they do not come into the house, they have sufficient sheltered areas that allow them to lie down on a clean, dry surface.

It is interesting to note how Mr. M. allowed his earlier dogs (potcakes) to roam, but his current dogs (pure-bred or "mixed" breed[22]) are not allowed to roam. Further, while his previously owned females bred, he soon prevented the current one from having pups. Despite his "love" for his pets, Mr. M. finds it difficult to determine when his pets should be put down and his preference would be for them to "just die," an action mentioned by some in the perception studies; he gives the impression that the animal's suffering must be clear before he would part with his pet.

His primary reason for having his dogs as "pets" is that they provide an outlet for affection ("love"). Although he also makes the analogy of dogs/pups being like children, the dogs have no place inside the house. This may be understandable due to the physical limitations of the house, which is clearly home to many adults and children, and so there is no additional space to accommodate two large dogs. However, Mr. M. clearly considers that the number of dogs one can own is constrained by the size of the yard, and so he appears to regard the yard as being the place where dogs are kept.

Although Mr. M. feels that the laws regarding animal ownership should be "harsher" with higher fines, he, himself a policeman, ignores the legal requirement to register ownership. It would appear that the dog license law is not perceived to be important, even to those who want the law enforced. This unwillingness to license the dogs is consistent with the historical actions of dog owners.

General

These two contrasting interviews provide a context for the findings of the resident perception studies and suggest that some of the responses in the perception studies should not be interpreted at face value. They also show that much valuable information can be obtained by visiting people's homes and comparing owners' answers to the conditions under which animals are kept. Although it is important to obtain people's perceptions, it is essential to check them so that the effectiveness of actions or accuracy of statements can be assessed. For example, in our perception study 43% of owners said that they take their pets to the veterinarian "when needed," but the level of health care this provides could be so low as to effectively mean "never"; thus only 34% of owners may be providing adequate health care for their pets. In terms of health care, Mr. M. might be regarded as being in the "top" third of pet owners, and Miss F. in the "bottom" two-thirds.

These interviews also suggest that more than the admitted 53% of households may feed roaming dogs, so such a figure should be viewed as a minimum value.[23] It is clear that there is a discrepancy between what people intend to do and the actual outcome of their actions. Although Miss F. does not mean to feed roaming dogs (and vermin) she does because of the way she feeds her dogs. As with other aspects of human behaviour, her convenience comes first, and the wider (may be major) consequences of her actions to others come second.[24]

These observations highlight some of the issues raised in connection with roaming dogs and garbage below. It is easy to see why the roaming dog population is able to survive on a diet of garbage and food scraps when people put out food that is accessible to all dogs. It also suggests that if such behaviour is widespread, a major component behind the increasing dog population is the increasing number of households. As the number of households increases, more food is made available to roaming dogs, and so a larger number of such dogs can be supported.

If dogs were restrained, there would be fewer dogs seen roaming; however, if people such as Mrs. F. confine their dogs to a stock-proof yard, it is still important that the dogs be neutered to prevent breeding. While fencing in dogs will remove them from the streets, it will not stop them breeding; thus fencing in without neutering will not reduce the dog population. Unwanted pups from unplanned litters from owned dogs can be abandoned and so owned pups can be transferred to the unowned, roaming population. (The repercussions of abandonment are in Chapter 10.) This is one example of where at least two dog-control policy measures must be implemented simultaneously if the objective of reducing the roaming dog population is to be achieved.

Fencing in will reduce contact between dogs and so should reduce the incidence of communicable diseases, such as sexually transmitted ones. As a result, the health of fenced-in dogs could be expected to be better than if the dogs were allowed to roam, an observation consistent with one of Miss F.'s. and from our data (see Chapter 10).

Both interviewees consider that they look after their pets well, even though their level of care might still give cause for concern. This is probably just another example of self-deception and a manifestation of the fact that we often do not judge ourselves by the standards we set others. All dog owners who claim to love their pets would consider themselves to look after their pets well (for example, how many "loving" parents would admit to not looking after their children well?). They would never admit, or even notice, that they neglected an object of love or acted in anything other than what they perceive to be its best interests. It is notable that both owners feed their dogs almost identical food and quantities. This suggests that either or both owners consider feeding as the single most important aspect of good pet care. Their actions give the impression that not to feed a dog would be considered very poor pet care. This view also accounts for the fact that people still feed roaming dogs even though they suffer from the "nuisances" which such animals cause, and is consistent with many people feeding animals they do not own. Such people see themselves as caring or being kind to these animals. Such actions could account for the fact that few under-fed dogs are seen.

The lack of enforcement of the laws concerning dogs has been observed as far back as Powles and beyond. This study shows that people are ignorant on the laws with respect to dogs.[25] If it is convenient to the owner to let the dog roam, this happens. Miss F., although a dog lover, sees no requirement to comply with the dog license law and does not even know how to license the dogs. Mr. M. wants more law enforcement, but apparently inconvenient laws, such as licensing dogs, can be ignored. Few car owners would admit to not knowing how to license a car (or that it was unlicensed) because the police enforce the law on car licensing. The police visibly enforce this law at the beginning of each month when old car licenses expire. While laws concerning dogs are rarely enforced, there is little incentive for owners to comply with them.[26]

Both interviews indicate a more limited level of human-dog interaction than found in some Western societies. A "happy" dog is said to require human affection. Reasons for keeping an animal as a "pet" include:

- Something to care for
- Something to touch
- Something to keep one busy
- A focus of attention
- A reason for exercise
- Something to make one feel safer[27]

The level of human-dog interaction in our interviews is reflected with most dogs being kept "in the yard," and is consistent with the findings of the pet attachment study. If many yard-dogs have fleas etc., or appear dirty, this makes them less likely to be invited inside the house. We suggest that the level of affection given a dog decreases as it grows from pup to dog[28] (also mentioned in Stubbs' song; see page 19). As the level of interaction decreases, affection further decreases. The dog is still fed (as it is perceived to be cruel not to do so), yet cost, time and trouble result in the dog's not visiting a veterinarian regularly, and as the dog starts to look sicker, the level of interaction spirals down again. This interaction may be further reduced if the animal is a potcake, as indicated in the focus groups. The limited interaction between dogs and humans makes roaming dogs shy and wary of humans, and this has resulted in their being termed "wild" in the press.[29] In the Turks and Caicos Islands, potcakes are often called "feral" or "wild," as they are "uncared for"[30]—but then if these animals have no interaction with humans, it is strange that they only like cooked food.[31] Such terminology, with its emotive overtones, only helps to discourage interaction.

The companionable aspect of dog ownership was noted in both interviews. Companionable bonds can only be made when there is close contact and interaction between dog and owner. In a person's early development, interaction with an animal teaches them much which can be applied to later life; hence, the link between animal cruelty and crime.[32] When dogs are kept outside, such bonds are hard to form. When pet care is limited, animals can soon die, and so strong bonds between owner and pet are difficult to make. In the pet attachment study "older"[33] people were no more attached to their pets than younger people. Older people, particularly those who live alone, can derive much pleasure and personal benefit from pets.[34] As human populations age and family units become less stable, pet ownership can become more important, as pets provide company and interest which were once given by family members caring for the elderly. Changes in current pet care might allow the companionable aspects of pet ownership to be further exploited to the benefit of both the owners and pets.

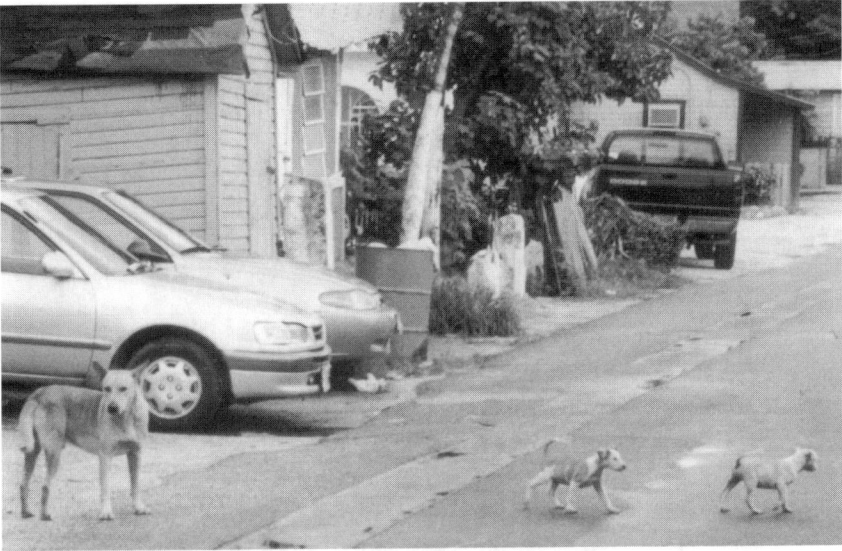

Roaming dogs need to learn to be streetwise at an early age. The harshness of street life constrains the growth of the roaming dog population.

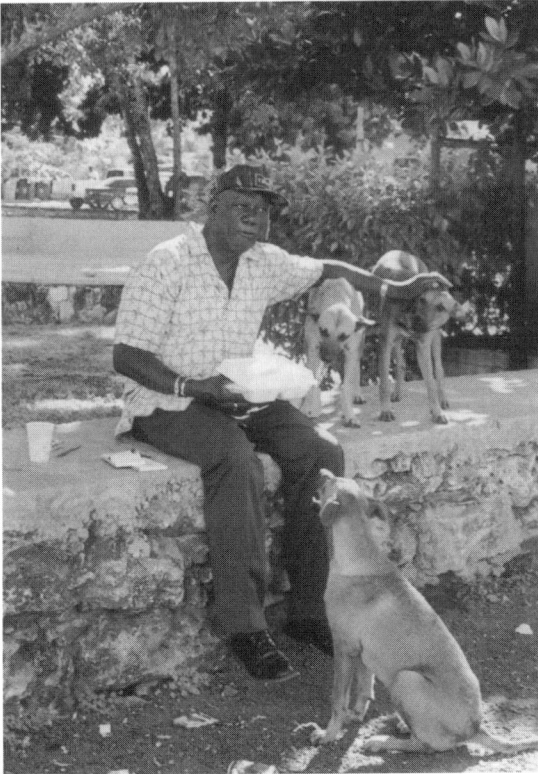

Many residents feed dogs they do not own, as they feel sorry for the "hungry" dogs. These dogs may be hungry, but clearly they are not starving. Feeding roaming dogs illustrates the ambivalent attitudes residents have towards roaming dogs.

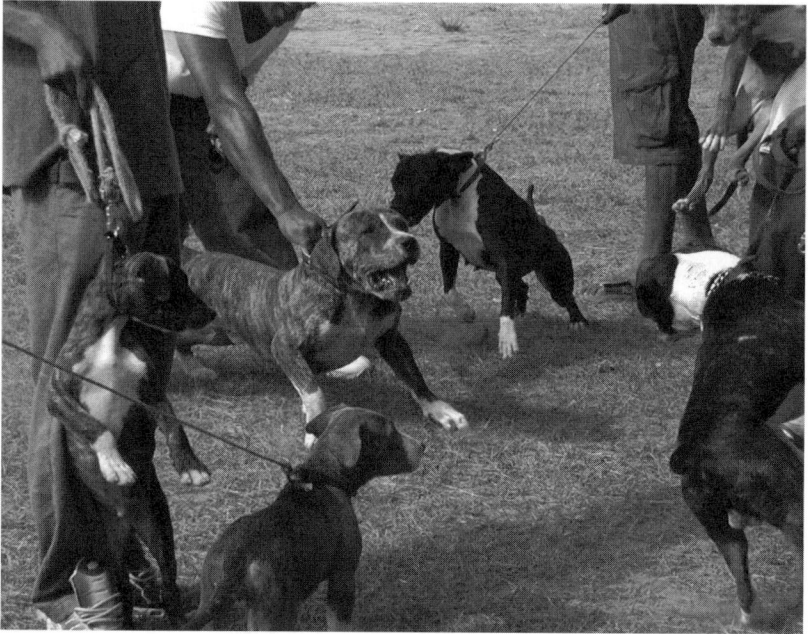

Pit bull types are commonly associated with young males. Pit bulls have been implicated in all the fatal dog attacks in New Providence.

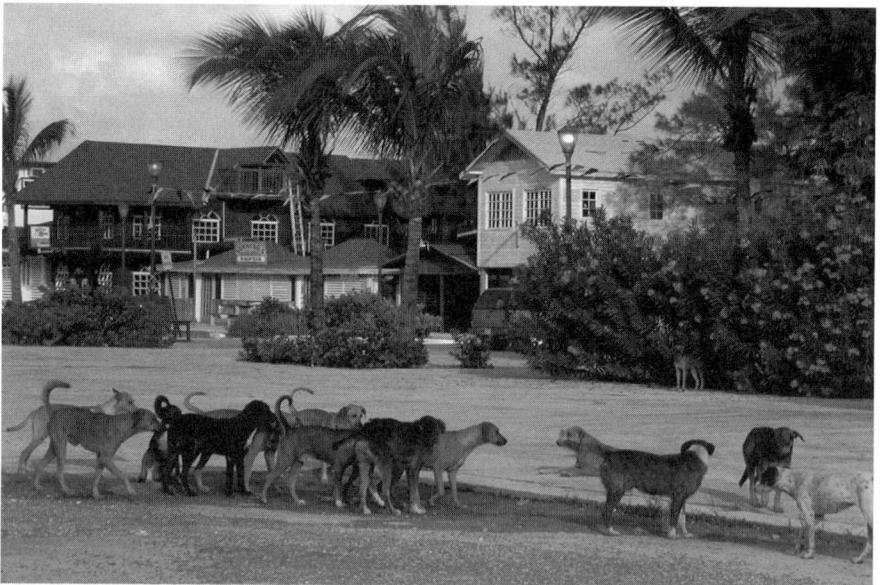

Large packs of dogs (this pack had about 24 in total) not only show the variability within the potcake population but can make humans fearful for their safety.

8

Roaming Dogs

> As for the curs which roam about the streets at night,
> they are of no use to God or man ...[1]

As indicated in the Introduction, free-roaming dogs have "always" been a feature of New Providence's environment and they have "always" been considered a "nuisance" or "problem." This situation has arisen despite it being illegal to allow dogs to roam unattended:

> It shall be lawful ... to seize any ... dog [licensed or unlicensed] ... found in any highway, or other place of public resort between the hours of ten o'clock in the night and six o'clock in the morning unattended by the owner ...[2]

Prior to 1998, the topic of "stray" dogs had been the subject of much speculation. Press articles had usually either been written by veterinarians, animal rights activists or were reports of politicians' or government rhetoric,[3] and so had been agenda-driven. The speculation and misrepresentation typical of issues surrounding this emotive topic can be illustrated by attempts to quantify the number of free-roaming dogs. Government awareness of the nuisance had resulted in a committee on stray dogs in 1996. An estimate of 45,000 owned dogs was mentioned at a meeting of this committee, and by 1998 this was being reported in the press as the population of free-roaming dogs![4] Misinformation about roaming dogs is still circulated and repeated, in particular as it relates to their breeding ability. Typically, the public is informed how one female dog can produce thousands of other dogs during her lifetime.[5] Unsupported assumptions about the behaviour of owners are also made. For example, a neuter programme was aimed at male owners, based on the assumption that male owners are less likely than female owners to neuter their dogs.[6] The targeting of male owners in a Bahamian context is an example of uncritically transferring observations from elsewhere and assuming that they can be applied here.[7]

The terms "cur" or "stray" dog have been typically applied to free-roaming dogs.[8] These words have been used because it seems that people have considered dogs seen on the streets as being unowned, although they are aware that owned dogs also roam. Use of the word "stray" also seems to suggest that the dogs themselves, rather than humans, are responsible for the perceived "stray dog problem." In recent years, however, the term "wild"[9] has been used to describe these animals, which adds further, unsubstantiated nuances about the characteristics of roaming dogs. We use the term "roaming" to refer to all dogs that roam unattended, irrespective of their legal ownership status. Most roaming dogs are potcakes, but we also see pedigree and pedigree-type dogs, dogs with collars and dogs with docked tails roaming,[10] findings consistent with the observation that owned (or at least once owned) dogs also roam.[11] We take the view that all unowned dogs roam, but of course not all owned dogs roam.

Simple arithmetic (using figures in Tables 10.3 and 10.16) indicates that if 20% of 73,200 dogs roam (or about 20,000 dogs), then almost all the "unowned" dogs (11,100) could be owned, which reinforces the view previously expressed by a veterinarian that owners should restrain their pets.[12] The inability of owners to restrict their pets to their premises, together with a lack of proper identification, means that it is hard to distinguish between owned and unowned dogs which roam. This confusion was illustrated in a newspaper picture of six roaming dogs which were described as "wild," yet at least two of the dogs in the photograph had collars, which shows that they certainly had had owners, even if they were not currently owned.[13] The inability to identify owners of roaming dogs hinders enforcement of laws concerning dogs.

Our 1998 "perception study" was the first attempt to take the debate about free-roaming dogs to the public and get its input with respect to attitudes and actions towards both owned and unowned dogs from a cross-section of society.

Composition of the free-roaming dog population

Casual observation of the roaming dog population reveals that it consists almost exclusively of "potcakes," although some owned "breed"[14] dogs are seen roaming. In our photographic capture-recapture study in Abaco, no recognizable purebred dogs were seen in 199 photographed dogs.[15] This suggests that, statistically, potcakes make up at least 98.5% of the roaming population.[16] As "breed" dogs interact with roaming dogs, "potcake mixes" are being seen; for example, a "shepherd potcake mix"[17] and "pitcakes," a pit bull–potcake mix.[18] Although relatively few pure-breed dogs roam, they appear to be more frightening to residents than potcakes:

> It is frightening to walk past some homes and have a big *Akita-dog* or a *Great Dane* come into the street barking at you, not to mention the savage *Pitbull* dogs that are *not* kept locked in their yards.[19]

Age and weights of roaming dogs

The Animal Control Unit has made available information on the sex, age and weight of eleven roaming dogs. A summary of the results is given in Table 8.1.

Table 8.1: Summary of median age, weight and breed characteristics of free-roaming dogs processed by the Animal Control Unit, Nassau.

	Age (years)	Weight (kg)	Sample size
Male "breed"	2.5	26.2	1
Female "breed"	2.5	20.3	1
Male potcakes	3.0	17.6	4
Female potcakes	1.5	13.1	5
All "breed"	2.5	23.3	2
All potcakes	1.5	16.7	9
All dogs	2.5	17.2	

The sample size is small, so only tentative observations can be made; females appear to have a lower average age than males, and they also appear to be smaller in size than males. "Breed" dogs appear to be heavier than potcakes, even though the "breed" dogs were surrendered or caught after being abandoned[20] and so were usually in poor condition. The average age, 2.5 years, is in line with that reported in other roaming dog populations.[21]

The weights for these dogs are higher than those seen in other free-roaming dog populations, which suggests that food is not a factor limiting their welfare.[22] The weights for the potcakes are in line with that laid down by the "potcake standard" of the Bahamas Kennel Club. This observation is consistent with the common observation that relatively few thin roaming dogs are seen in New Providence. (The availability of food for roaming dogs is discussed in the section "Garbage and Free-Roaming Dogs.")

Breeding patterns of free-roaming dogs

The Government's Animal Control Unit receives and collects unwanted dogs. Almost all the animals processed by the Unit are potcakes, although some neglected purebred dogs are also seen. Animals coming into the Animal Control Unit are primarily, but not exclusively, roaming dogs. Examination of the number of dogs and puppies processed by the Animal Control Unit over a three-year period (1997–1999) showed one peak in the number of puppies during the year. This indicates that roaming dogs do not breed twice a year, because such a breeding pattern would result in two peaks (Figure 8.1). This finding shows that the free-roaming population is unable to reproduce as often as believed. The idea that free-roaming dogs breed prolifically is probably due to the fact that they breed all year round. Figure 8.1 shows that while potcakes in general breed all year round, the same potcakes do not breed every six months. The existence of a single peak in number of potcake puppies has also been noted by the owners of shops in New Providence and Abaco that operate adoption programmes. The inability of free-roaming dogs to breed often has been observed in other roaming populations.[23] However, the misconception about the ability of roaming dogs to increase their numbers still persists in The Bahamas.[24] One group of (legally) owned but unlicensed, roaming dogs appears to have failed to increase its size during a two-year period, despite several litters of puppies being born.[25]

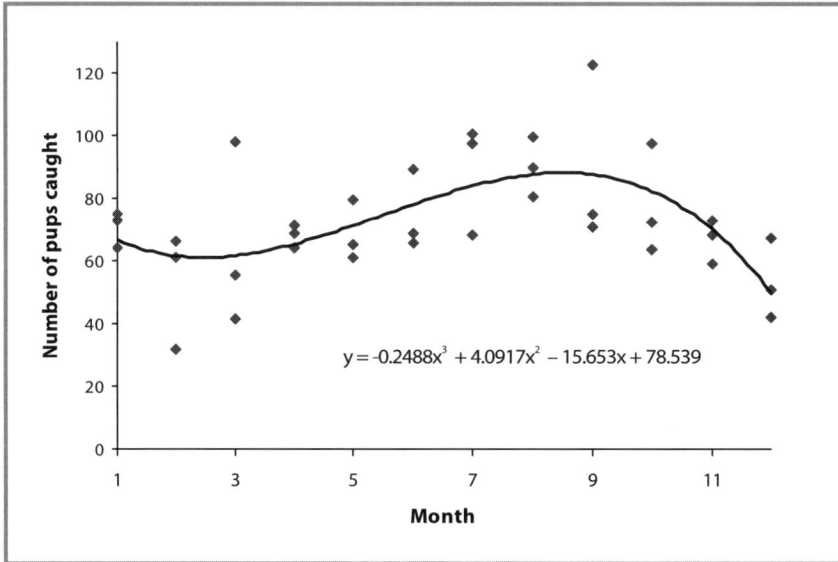

Figure 8.1: Pattern of puppy catches by the Animal Control Unit, 1997–1999, Nassau.
Catch figures adjusted for the number of adult dogs caught. Reproduced with permission from Fielding, W. J. and Mather, J. (2001). Dog ownership in the West Indies: A case study from The Bahamas. *Anthrozoös* 14(2): 72–80.

These are very important observations, as they counter the myth that potcakes breed "all the time."[26] Clearly they do breed throughout the year, but this is distinct from individuals breeding "all the time." Thus there is a major constraint on the growth of the roaming dog population, which explains why the island is not overrun with roaming dogs, despite the warnings of some animal welfare groups.

Again these observations point to the need for a sustained national/public education programme based on local facts. They also highlight the need to assess foreign information from a local perspective, rather than simply assuming that it applies to The Bahamas. Uncritical use of foreign information can result in the public being mislead rather than being educated.

Litter size of free-roaming dogs

As yet we have little information on this. Although it is clear that the breeding interval of roaming dogs exceeds six months, the number of puppies that survive from a litter to breeding age is less clear. One group of about four owned, roaming dogs, on a building site in the west of the island, has been observed periodically from 1999 to early 2003. From three litters, only two puppies appear to have reached breeding age after natural and human culling (at least two were poisoned, one dog was run over, one appeared to wander off and get detached from the group, and some puppies were taken by residents to the Bahamas Humane Society). This would suggest that the survival rate to breeding age is low. A litter born in early 2002 appears to have had just one survivor (from at least five) still on the site.

Health of free-roaming dogs

Ninety-five percent of free-roaming dogs have heartworm (*Dirofilariasis*) by the time they are one year old.[27] This means that the life expectancy of such animals is about three years.[28] A visual inspection of dogs at the Animal Control Unit showed that 70% of the dogs were suffering from disease. Venereal tumors, hook worm (*Ancylostoma caninum*) and other parasites are reported by veterinarians to be common in the roaming dog population.[29] Poor health might be one of the constraints on the breeding ability of roaming dogs noted above.

Constraints on the free-roaming population and their effects

The population growth of the roaming dog population is limited by breeding frequency, poor health, deaths by cars and poisoning etc., and removals by the Animal Control Unit.[30] If we assume that the rate of growth of the roaming dog population is linked to the growth rate of the number of households[31] (because so many householders feed roaming dogs; see Table 8.2), we can derive a "balance sheet" showing the relative importance of selected factors influencing the dog population. If we assume that the mortality rate is double that seen in the owned dog population,[32] this allows us to impute a birth figure. The balance sheet clearly shows that the free-roaming dog population is maintained by recruits from the owned dog population, i.e. abandoned dogs. This important finding is revisited in our discussion of Table 10.16.

Regrettably, these observations concerning the limitations on the ability of roaming dogs to breed continue to be overlooked by well-meaning animal activists who frighten the public with the unlikely arithmetic that an unspayed dog can be responsible for thousands of offspring during her lifetime.[33] Such scaremongering is unlikely to endear roaming dogs (generally potcakes) to the general public and diverts attention from the role the public can play in controlling the dog population.

Residents' perceptions of free-roaming dogs

One of the major concerns about free-roaming dogs is their number. The media often suggests that the "stray dog" population is growing, without stating the basis for the statement,[34] or that the "potcake menace will not go away."[35] How can the perception that the roaming dog population is increasing be explained in the absence of a monitoring programme? Is the activity of roaming dogs such that their numbers can appear to be greater than they really are? Much has been written about the behaviour of roaming dogs,[36] all of which could be expected to apply to the roaming dog population of New Providence. Both increased temperatures and increased human activity reduce the number of dogs seen on the street. Both these factors could affect people's perception of the dog numbers. In addition, observations along one street in Nassau from September to June show that the number of roaming dogs is related to sunrise time (Figure 8.2).[37] Although these observations were taken at about the same time each day (around 7.45 a.m. local time on school days only[38]), it is clear that the number of dogs is related to sunrise (at –5 GMT), despite considerable day-to-day variation. Thus, it is understandable why residents could get the impression that the dog population is increasing when in fact it may be virtually static. Figure 8.2 also indicates how difficult it is assess long-term changes in roaming dog populations. Comparable observations would have to be taken at the same time each year, or at least similar sunrise times, to assess changes in the roaming dog population.

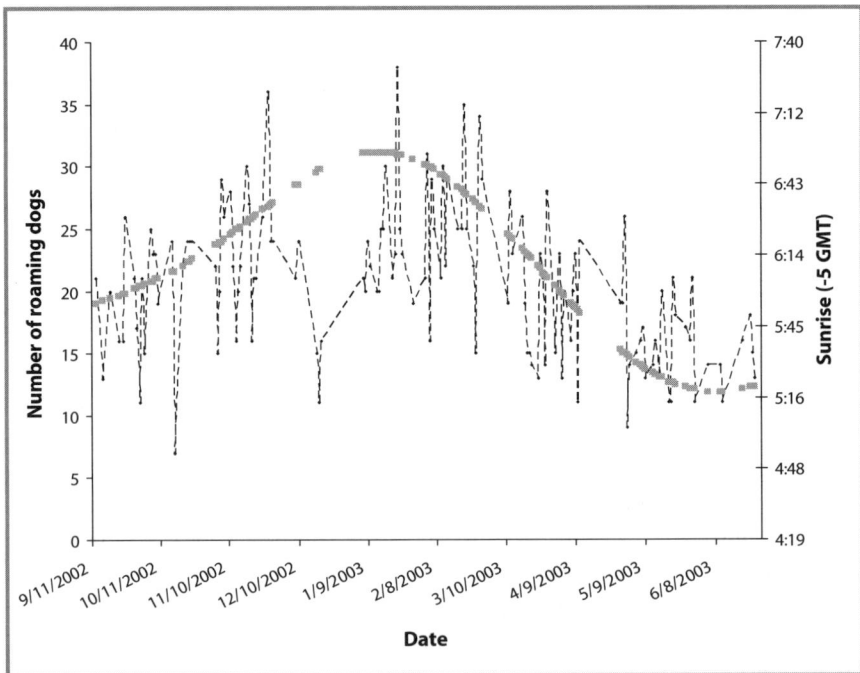

Figure 8.2: Numbers of roaming dogs seen along Kemp Road, and sunrise times, September 2002 to June 2003.

The majority of residents agree that The Bahamas does indeed suffer from a "stray dog problem," but this does not mean that draconian measures to reduce the free-roaming population would be acceptable. There is a ground-swell of good-will towards free-roaming animals despite the nuisance such animals cause residents. This attitude is consistent with the ambivalent view that we have already seen society has towards potcakes. From Table 8.2, 90% in our study thought that The Bahamas has a "stray dog problem."[39] In Bain Town, 97% (of 35 respondents) thought that roaming dogs were a hazard to society, compared with 40% (of 35 respondents) in Yamacraw (p<0.001).[40] These differences again show local variation in the islandwide perception of the nuisance of roaming dogs.

Good-will towards potcakes was exhibited by over half those we interviewed who feed dogs which they do not own; indeed, over half of those who personally suffered the nuisances of roaming dogs still fed them.[41] In the study of Bain Town and Yamacraw, 77% and 66%, respectively, of respondents fed dogs in the community.[42] Reasons for feeding dogs which people do not claim to own include: "The food is there," "the neighbours do not look after them," "they are hungry." Our respondents fed a mean of 2.4 (se=0.24) roaming dogs each. However, people who feed roaming dogs do not necessarily feed them every day. In another study, only 56% of residents who said that they fed roaming dogs had actually fed a roaming dog the day before the interview.[43] Applying this level of frequency in New Providence would mean that 18,000 roaming dogs might be fed each day. However, it should be noted that some of these unowned dogs might be community-owned dogs, rather than individually owned dogs, or the same dog fed by several people. (See the section on community owned dogs below.) Tourists also feed roaming dogs. At popular tourist locations, such as Fort Fincastle and the water tower, Prince George Wharf, and Bay Street, many roaming dogs appear to thrive on the presence of tourists. Thus, it should be noted that residents are not alone in making food available to roaming dogs.[44]

Although people "run dogs" from their yard, they rarely take stronger measures than throwing a stone,[45] despite the dogs' being a nuisance. Most interviewees clearly wanted roaming dogs dealt with in a humane way. Although euthanasia was commonly proposed, this was usually suggested for sick dogs; people wanted healthy animals adopted or allowed to live out their lives. Any suggestion that roaming dogs should be simply killed would clearly not meet with the approval of the majority. In fact, some people (2%) felt that the dogs should be simply left alone. There may be important community variations as to how people want the "problem" solved. For example, in Bain Town, 25% of respondents wanted the dogs killed, whereas no respondent in Yamacraw suggested this.[46] However, these views contrast with reports of the Animal Control Unit being prevented from catching dogs in Bain Town,[47] and so highlight the diversity of views even within a small community towards animal control.

The tolerance of residents to free-roaming dogs can be illustrated by our own experience. Roaming dogs were frequenting the grounds surrounding WF's office. It was not until there were six dogs, some of which started to bark at staff, that action was taken to have them removed. Studies elsewhere have reported a similar tolerance of residents to lone roaming dogs, but dislike of packs of dogs.[48]

Table 8.2: Some attitudes towards free-roaming and unowned ("stray") dogs in New Providence, The Bahamas.

Attitudes towards unowned animals		Number responding
Feel sympathetic towards "stray" dogs	93%	303
Think there is a "stray" dog problem in The Bahamas	90%	299
Have "strays" in their neighborhood	77%	299
Think "strays" are a health hazard "in general"	65%	284
Feed dogs they do not own	53%	296
Have adopted a "stray" cat or dog	41%	306
Have garbage spilt by "strays"*	34%	306
Want "stray" population controlled by adoption*	34%	298
Want "stray" population controlled by "putting to sleep"*	32%	298
Have been bitten (or had a family member) bitten by a "stray"	25%	306
Want "strays" controlled by "housing/ confining"*	21%	298
Suffer from barking "strays"	18%	306
Want the "stray" population left alone*	2%	298
Consider "strays" to be a personal nuisance	46%	306
Suffer a personal nuisance: garbage spilt*	78%	135
Suffer a personal nuisance from barking "strays"	41%	135
Suffer a personal nuisance: dog faeces	33%	135
Suffer a personal nuisance: dogs mating	9%	135
Think "strays" are a personal health hazard	11%	135

Not all questionnaires were fully completed. Some questions were only asked to the relevant sub-population of interviewees.
*Respondents were allowed multiple responses to questions concerning nature of nuisances and method of population control.
Expanded, and reproduced with permission, from Fielding, W. J. and Mather, J. (2000). *Journal of Applied Animal Welfare Science* 3(4): 305–319.

The scattering of garbage and barking at night were the two most commonly reported problems attributed to roaming dogs.[49] However, attributing barking at night to unowned dogs is mistaken, as they are generally shy and do not seek to attract attention. As will be seen later, it is the many dogs owned to protect households that probably bark most. In fact, we have seen owned dogs bark furiously on "their" property or territory, but these same dogs are extremely quiet when roaming in a neighbour's lot. This shyness was also observed by Powles in 1888 (see page 8 above). However, we do note that roaming dogs can be noisy when groups of dogs find a female in heat or are involved in chase behaviour. When a female is in heat, the response of dogs can be such as to make them a hazard to traffic and a nuisance to residents.

Only a third of respondents who suffered from the nuisance of roaming dogs mentioned dog faeces. We feel that many people are unaware of the potential public health issues associated with dog faeces and urine, probably because they are accustomed to the presence of dog faeces. We are unaware of any study of dog faeces in New Providence, so the health risks associated with it have yet to be evaluated.

Garbage and free-roaming dogs

As Table 8.2 indicates, the most commonly reported nuisance of roaming dogs is that they tip over garbage.[50] This action not only makes the streets unsightly, but also makes the contents readily available for other animals, in particular small rodents that might not otherwise gain access to the contents of bins.

Dogs tip over the bins because they are looking for food, and because the bins are stored in such a way that dogs have access to them. Interestingly enough, households which complain about their garbage being scattered by dogs are breaking the law,[51] as the law requires garbage to be stored so that it does not become scattered! The law on this issue is enforced more rigorously than the regulations regarding dogs, partly because it is easier to prove ownership of garbage than of untagged dogs.[52]

Even well-fed dogs are always on the lookout for more food, so it is difficult to determine how hungry scavenging dogs actually are. Further, as many people feed roaming dogs, it is hard to determine the importance to their survival of the food that they find in the bins. A case study of the contents of WF's garbage (from a family of four) showed that enough food was thrown out between the weekly garbage collections to feed one dog. Table 8.3 shows that about 12 kg of rubbish are thrown out each week and about 3 kg, or 25%, are edible.

This result agreed with data obtained by consultants gathering information on garbage in general in New Providence.[53] Thus, it would appear that the food in domestic garbage alone would be enough to feed as many as 20,000 dogs. Even if the food in the bins is not an important component of the dogs' diet, the availability of food encourages dogs into people's yards; they then cause a nuisance and so invite inhumane actions from annoyed householders.

Free-roaming dogs may have access to around 20,000–40,000 garbage bins (i.e., bins that are not properly stored), which could contain between 3.4 and 6.8 million litres of garbage each week. The case study data suggest that this garbage alone could provide enough food to sustain a population of 17,500 unowned dogs.[54] In addition, we estimate that some 26,000 households feed free-roaming dogs. Some residents claimed to feed these dogs in the hope that the animals will not tip over their garbage bins. This seems optimistic, because those who fed unowned dogs encouraged dogs to visit their yard.[55] The availability of food from garbage and handouts can also encourage owned dogs to roam, particularly if owners do not feed their pets regularly. These observations suggest that there is a considerable amount of food accessible to free-roaming dogs. The result of residents feeding dogs that they do not own and the availability of domestic and commercial garbage is that relatively few thin free-roaming dogs are seen[56] and that these dogs are relatively large (Table 8.1).

When people see thin roaming dogs, lack of food is probably not the cause of their appearance. There is clearly an abundant supply of food for roaming dogs, from handouts to leftover food put out for owned dogs to food in accessible garbage. Consequently, when people see thin dogs, they are probably seeing sick dogs; their thinness a result of ill-health rather than starvation. If this is so, it highlights the inadequacy of the care that people offer when they only feed dogs which they do not own.

Table 8.3: Average weight of garbage items, according to category (average of two weeks) from a "richer" four person-household in New Providence.

Source	Weight (kg)	% of total weight
Glass, clean	2.35	20%
Other cardboard/paper/plastic	2.08	17%
Cardboard/paper/plastic, soiled with food	2.08	17%
Glass, soiled with food/drink	1.22	10%
Fruit, fruit skins, etc.	0.95	8%
Uncooked vegetables and peelings, etc.	0.77	6%
Cooked meat/bones	0.55	5%
Metal tins, etc. soiled with food/drink	0.48	4%
Flowers, plants, etc.	0.46	4%
Bread, cake, etc.	0.32	3%
Other metal	0.18	2%
Eggs, egg shells	0.14	1%
Cloth	0.11	1%
Cooked vegetables	0.10	1%
Rice, potatoes (cooked), etc.	0.09	1%
Cheese	0.04	0%
Cooked fish/bones	0.00	0%
Uncooked fish/bones	0.00	0%
Uncooked meat/bones	0.00	0%
Newspapers, etc.	0.00	0%
Total	11.92	100%

Average number of 49 litre garbage bags used/week: 5; approximate total volume: 245 litres.
"Richer" is defined to be household income over $20,000 per year.

People seem unaware that food put out for dogs is also accessible to other creatures, particularly invasive species such as pigeons, ring neck doves, rats, mice, cockroaches and flies. Thus, people who feed free-roaming dogs can also encourage increases in the populations of rats, etc.[57] These pests almost certainly pose a greater threat to public health than dogs, and their presence, particularly of rats in tourist areas, has resulted in front-page newspaper headlines.[58] Increasingly, invasive birds are also becoming a nuisance in tourist locations where garbage is readily accessible.

Current government policy towards low-cost housing schemes excludes secure garbage storage areas,[59] making it harder for poorer people to properly store garbage. The percentage of food in household garbage increases as income level increases, from

9.2% to 14.4% from "low" to "high" income groups. Thus, unless people change their ways, as Bahamians become richer, more and more food will be available to dogs in garbage. While the correct storage of garbage will not stop dogs roaming, denying them access to garbage should divert dogs from residential areas, which should result in the animals being less of a nuisance to the community.

It should be noted that dogs can catch *Giardia* or *Cryprsporidium* infections from diapers.[60] Thus, the irresponsible storage of human garbage can be a health hazard to dogs. Both human and dog health are threatened by garbage which is tipped over.

There are, of course, other sources of waste food to which dogs have access: for example, garbage thrown in roadside bushes, etc. (23% food); waste food from hotels/restaurants, supermarkets, etc. (38% and 23% respectively) and of course rubbish dumps, etc.[61] Not surprisingly, in a tourist-based economy, the most important of these, in actual quantities, is food from hotels/restaurants and, obviously, dumps. Due to the large number of tourists, the quantity of garbage on the island is further increased by what the visitors consume locally and import. However, overall, we feel that given its scale—second only to hotels/restaurants etc. and its *widespread* availability—domestic garbage is the most important and difficult issue to address with regard to sources of food for unowned free-roaming dogs and their interaction with humans.

Roaming dogs as a health hazard

Probably as a response to media reports discussing roaming dogs and rabies,[62] residents consider roaming dogs to be a health hazard. Many newspaper reports, often written by veterinarians, have described the potential disorders that humans can catch from dogs in addition to being bitten.[63] This fear has taken root despite the experience, still common today, of roaming dogs avoiding close contact with humans. Although most people interviewed were concerned about roaming dogs as a health hazard, the fear was greatest amongst non-dog owners (70% of 161 replies) rather than dog owners (54% of 143 replies, p=0.01),[64] which indicates that the non-owning group may either not own dogs because of this fear, or ownership has given owners a more realistic understanding of the risk of dogs to their health.

Although 25% of respondents had been bitten or knew of relations bitten by "stray" dogs, such dogs might have been owned roaming dogs, as owned dogs are more likely to bite than unowned ones. (Health issues and dog bites are considered in greater detail in Chapters 15 and 16.)

Community-owned dogs

Traditional Caribbean houses are often unfenced[65] and in less affluent areas neighbours often share yards. While no individual household may claim to own the dogs, all the households tolerate the presence of the animals or consider the dogs as belonging there. Residents will usually have varying levels of commitment to the animals, with no defined responsibilities as to who tends them. While households will probably ensure that food and water are available to the dogs on a regular basis, there will be no guarantee that the animals will be fed each day. If the dog is a potcake, as is likely, the animal will probably not be given any health care or be neutered, as this would incur a clear financial cost. These animals would almost certainly not be confined, even if there is a fence around part or all of the yard. This social environment may help to explain why 70% of poorer people (those households earning $20,000 per year or less) compared to 46% of richer households (those earning over $20,000 per year) feed roaming dogs. A study of 117 students[66] found that 34% of respondents considered community dogs to be kept "acceptably" even though 51% of respondents reported seeing community dogs being allowed to roam and only 30% saw such dogs confined. Such roaming dogs are potential recruits to the unowned roaming dog population.

An interesting subgroup of community-owned dogs includes Collins. He, like others, is fed and given friendship by staff in their workplace. Such people include watchmen, who may welcome a companion at night and hope the dog would offer them some sort of protection; and "lunch ladies" who take pity on the animals and feed them on someone else's premises. These owners are protective of the dogs ("Why do you want to take his picture?") and the dogs appear to inhabit workplaces with the tacit approval of the employers. The College of The Bahamas cares for several potcakes ("College dogs") which roam the campus, and one of them was even featured on the College's 2003 calendar.[67]

For these reasons, in general, we consider community dogs as roaming dogs, although they are owned in the legal sense. Such dogs are probably included in the number of dogs that residents reported as feeding yet not owning, because they do not feel that they personally own the animals.[68]

While we have not made any attempt to identify the size of the community-owned dog population, community dogs will be most common in the poorer areas of the island, where communal yards are most often seen. Their distribution may be reflected in the variation of roaming numbers in different areas of New Providence reported in Chapter 2.

Comments

As they recognize no boundaries, roaming dogs, usually potcakes, are seen from rich areas, such as Lyford Cay, to the poorer inner-city areas. It would seem from reports in the press that their presence on the streets is becoming increasingly unpopular,[69] but expectations that dog catching alone will reduce the roaming dog population are mistaken.[70] However, the actions of many residents result in the roaming dog population being supported and even encouraged to visit residential areas. While many people wish to have roaming dogs removed from the streets, others do not, which highlights the variation in attitudes towards roaming dogs and might explain why it has been such a difficult issue to address. The issue is further complicated by the fact that many owners allow their dogs to roam and think it cruel to confine dogs, and this underscores the importance of education in the long-term solution to reducing the number of dogs on the streets. It is clear that potcakes, as roaming dogs, share similarities with roaming dog populations elsewhere. The interaction of residents and roaming dogs and the perceptions of residents are also not unique to New Providence.[71] These similarities give The Bahamas the opportunity to utilize proven methods which will result in the long-term control of the number of roaming dogs.

9

Tourists and Roaming Dogs

> The dogs pulled [the tourist] to the ground and started biting her and dragging her. Doing her best to fend them off, she pulled herself into the water, where the dogs were unwilling to go. But every time the waves rolled out and left her exposed, the dogs would attack again.[1]

As has already been stated, tourism is a long-standing pillar of the economy. Consequently, anything which may detract from the tourism product is of grave concern. As has been pointed out earlier, tourists have been interacting with roaming dogs since at least the 1880s, when Drysdale saw roaming dogs in tourist areas. The presence of roaming dogs has resulted in a continuous stream of letters from tourists complaining about "pathetic, half starved stray dogs roaming" in Bay and Shirley streets "from dawn to dusk."[2] In the 1970s, two tourists even claimed that they had been bitten by "wild dogs" twice in five days.[3]

In the 1980s, a tourist brochure on potcakes was produced to encourage "endearment rather than endangerment" when tourists encountered them.[4] However, both the Bahamas Humane Society[5] and the Department of Agriculture[6] still receive letters from tourists complaining about roaming dogs. At one tourist location in Nassau we have seen over 24 dogs at a time, and lesser numbers are seen around various tourist attractions. Press reports have indicated that tourists are unsettled by seeing packs of roaming dogs, whereas residents are not.[7] We note, however, that roaming dogs in tourist spots can exhibit quite different behaviour compared to roaming dogs in residential areas. Dogs seen at the water tower, Prince George Wharf—where cruise ships dock—and near Paradise Island bridge are tamer and less wary of humans than roaming dogs elsewhere. This suggests that these dogs do not fear the presence of people or maltreatment, and need not act threateningly towards visitors or residents. The attack cited above is rare and regrettable, but given the fickleness of tourists, even one attack can have effects out of all proportion to the event.

Visitors may have both positive and negative impacts on the roaming dog population. They have made residents more aware of animal care, and when tourists adopt potcakes they provide positive publicity about pet welfare.[8] However, tourists and tourism-related industries can provide food for dogs, which can draw dogs to tourist locations and make those areas less attractive. Thus food and improper garbage disposal by tourist-related industries encourages the presence of roaming dogs in downtown Nassau and even in Rawson Square, site of the House of Assembly.[9] "Snow birds" (winter residents) sometimes feed "starving" roaming dogs, but these animals effectively become abandoned when they leave. Such actions can be expected to maintain the roaming dog population. However, on the positive side, some "snow birds" assist in neuter programmes, particularly in islands outside of New Providence.

In 2002, 4.37 million visitors came to the country,[10] and therefore the actions and reactions of tourists towards roaming dogs, which of course invariably means potcakes, are important. In a small-scale study of 39 tourists in New Providence, 28% remembered seeing roaming dogs, and 5% said that the presence of these dogs adversely affected their vacation.[11] This might mean that 200,000 visitors per year are "distressed" or "feared for their safety" or "felt that Bahamians neglect their dogs."[12] In other countries with important tourism industries, inhumane killing of roaming dogs has attracted negative publicity in the international media.[13] Consequently, although tourists may not want to see roaming dogs, they also expect the animals to be treated humanely.

The Bahamian Government, in its submission to the "Convention on Biological Diversity," links "benign development control of pests (rats, mice) and stray dogs" with tourism, which shows the importance to policy makers of the association between tourists and "stray dogs."[14] The Ministry of Tourism is also concerned that tourists and residents have different perspectives on roaming dogs. It can be expected that tourists judge the acceptability of roaming dogs against the norms of their cultures, and where these differ, Bahamians may be negatively judged. Tourists from countries with rabies may have a greater concern of catching that and other diseases than residents.[15]

The official slogan of the Bahamian tourism industry is "The Islands of The Bahamas—It just keeps getting better," which encourages high expectations of all aspects of a visit. Tourists can now report their holiday experiences on the Internet,[16] so any individual's experience can be shared with millions worldwide, in addition to friends and relations. Further, tourists interested in animal welfare, particularly if they are "activists," can also utilize the Internet to highlight pet issues beyond the borders of their own country.[17]

As most tourists (85%) who visit The Bahamas come from North America,[18] it is important for Bahamians to know how Americans view pets and how this may influence their perception of Bahamians and pet care in The Bahamas. Several differences between these two groups of owners are presented in Table 9.1. While such comparisons in themselves must be treated with caution, they may be useful in identifying possible areas of pet care which might cause concern to tourists. It is thought that tourists might be particularly sensitive to seeing roaming dogs while on vacation, as in a foreign study 35% of tourists "admitted to missing their pets more than anyone or anything when away on holiday" and 11% telephoned home to speak to their pets.[19]

Table 9.1: A comparison of selected aspects of dog ownership in The Bahamas and the United States.

	Bahamas	USA
Percentage of homes with dogs	43%	37%
Mean no. of dogs per household	2.6	1.4
Median age of dog (years)	3	5
Dogs which are pure-breds	<10%	62%
% taking dogs to the vet at least once a year	34%*	90%
% of dogs neutered	42%	66%

*Also includes cats. Data on The Bahamas from our studies. Data on the USA from Ralston Purina (2000). Op. cit.

A study of 439 adult tourists with US passports who were interviewed at popular tourist locations in and around Nassau attempted to discover the reactions of tourists towards roaming dogs. (American tourists were chosen because they make up the majority of tourists.)[20] Only if an interviewee had seen a roaming dog were reactions to roaming dogs solicited.

Thirty-three percent of the respondents were cruise ship passengers and the remainder were longer-stay visitors. Overall, 59% of the respondents were under 35 years of age and 50% were male. Overall, a visitor directly talked to a median of 15 people (range 0–2,000) about their vacation and 97% of respondents said they would either return to or recommend a vacation in The Bahamas to others.

Eighty-nine percent of tourists liked dogs and 49% currently owned dogs. Six percent were members of animal welfare groups and 14% had given money to an animal welfare group in the last 12 months.

Reactions to roaming dogs

Overall, 45% of respondents remembered seeing roaming dogs during their stay. Dogs were seen in all areas which tourists generally visit and in all areas where tourists were interviewed. Fifty percent of respondents (n=188) saw dogs in the noon-day hours, but dogs were seen at all times of the day. When tourists had noticed roaming dogs, their observations and reactions were obtained. A summary of their responses is listed in Table 9.2. Additional reactions are given in Table 9.3. Only one tourist made any complaint about the roaming dogs to a hotel employee. Sixty-six percent of respondents who saw roaming dogs thought that it was cruel, rather than kind, to let dogs roam. Of the 18 comments concerning the impact of the dogs on the vacation, only one was positive. All nine comments given as to how the presence of the dogs had altered the tourist's opinion of The Bahamas were negative. These comments included reactions such as "Bahamians are not kind," "Bahamians do not care," and "Not what was shown in the travel brochures."

Table 9.2: A summary of the main reaction of American tourists in New Providence to seeing roaming dogs (190 replies).

Main reaction	Response (%)
No reaction	40
Felt sorry for the dogs	26
Concerned for the dogs' safety	16
Pleased to see the dogs enjoying their freedom	9
Disgusted	4
Concerned for personal safety	3
Scared	2
Angry	0.5

Table 9.3: A summary of the observations and reactions of American tourists in New Providence to roaming dogs.

Observations	Response	Number responding
Modal time dogs were seen	Midday hours (51%)	189
Modal condition of dogs	"Fair" (40%)	196
Modal activity of the dogs	Walking (69%)	193
Reactions		
It is cruel to allow dogs to roam	66%	183
They might get sick from roaming dogs	28%	430
The Bahamas has a roaming dog problem	23%	188
The dogs had an impact on their visit	12%	192
Their view of The Bahamas was changed by seeing the dogs	8%	192
They felt scared or threatened	5%	190
They heard other tourists worried about roaming dogs	3%	427
They fed dogs	3%	193
They were bothered by dogs	3%	192
They saw other tourists bothered by dogs	1%	193

While no cruise ship passenger fed roaming dogs, 1% of all tourists did, and three of the five respondents who fed roaming dogs did so more than once.

Dog ownership and animal welfare characteristics of American tourists

Some characteristics of the tourists with respect to dog ownership and animal welfare were also obtained. These are summarized in Table 9.4.

Table 9.4: Dog ownership and animal welfare characteristics of American tourists visiting New Providence.

Dog ownership characteristics		Number responding
Like dogs	89%	429
Are dog owners	49%	429
Mean number of dogs owned	1.7 (se=0.06)	203
Modal source of last dog	breeder (33%)	212
Modal frequency of dog walks	daily (70%)	213
Owners celebrating their dog's birthday	55%	213
Animal welfare characteristics		
Gave money to an animal welfare group in last year	14%	426
Have a roaming dog problem where they live	7%	401
Member of an animal welfare group	6%	428

Six percent of tourists were members of animal welfare groups. If a tourist was a member of at least one animal welfare group, it was usually a humane group (85%, n=20), but 20% of that group were also members of People for the Ethical Treatment of Animals (or overall, just less than 1%). Although all the People for the Ethical Treatment of Animals members (n=3) saw roaming dogs, none of them were upset; two were concerned for the dogs' safety, and one felt sorry for them. None of the People for the Ethical Treatment of Animals members (n=4) would be upset to see animal control officers at work, a view consistent with their concern for the safety of the dogs.

Three tourists (0.7%), none of whom intended to return or recommend The Bahamas to others, appeared to have been adversely affected by the dogs, as they responded negatively to almost all the aspects of roaming dogs covered in the study. None of these were members of any animal welfare group but two were dog owners. Further, none of these three would object to seeing animal control officers at work.

A larger percentage of tourists were dog owners than was expected; tourists seemed to own more dogs than the "average" American dog owner, and are more likely to get their dogs from breeders and more likely to celebrate their dog's birthday.[21] Thus, tourists may be particularly aware of animal welfare, as 14% of them gave money to animal welfare groups, and their apparent preference for pure-bred dogs may make them more sensitive to potcakes than might be otherwise be the case.

As shown in Table 9.1, tourists can expect to have different views on dog ownership compared to Bahamians. Some differences may be due to tourists' owning fewer dogs and taking them to the veterinarian more frequently. The fact that only 7% of tourists have a roaming dog problem where they lived might make most tourists more conscious of seeing roaming dogs than otherwise. Over 65% of tourists thought it was cruel to allow dogs to roam, and so the sight of the dogs probably conveyed a negative image of dog owning in The Bahamas. This view of allowing dogs to roam as "cruel" contrasts with that of Bahamians, as 42% of them thought it cruel to confine dogs,[22] so this group would certainly allow their dogs to roam. Such differences in the views between tourists and Bahamians can lead to visitors thinking, rightly or wrongly, that Bahamians do not care for their pets.

Despite their pet owning background, many tourists did not notice the dogs, particularly if they were cruise ship passengers, and even when they did, most were unaffected by them. The observation that roaming dogs were seen by tourists in all the typical tourist locations and mainly in the noon-day hours probably reflects widespread occurrence of the dogs and the activities of tourists rather than any peculiarities in the activities of roaming dogs.[23]

Although only a small percentage of tourists did feed dogs, this could represent a large enough number of tourists (several hundred each day) to support the idea that tourists can prove to be an important source of food. Consequently, this action of the tourists may indeed help prop up the roaming dog population in tourist areas, or at least encourage them to frequent these spots and so make the dogs even more visible.

Although the presence of roaming dogs was generally viewed unfavorably, only one person actually complained, and 10% of tourists would be upset to see the dogs being captured by animal control officers. This reaction has important consequences for the implementation of dog population control measures at tourist locations. Thus, it is easy to conclude that tourists feel sorry for the dogs, rather than threatened, and a small core of tourists feel negatively towards Bahamians with regard to pet care (Table 9.2). Although only small numbers of tourists reacted adversely to seeing the dogs, a greater number said that they would be upset by seeing animal control officers catching dogs.[24] This tolerance/ambivalence towards to animals is similar to that shown by Bahamians; roaming dogs are a nuisance which is not liked, but people do not want the animals harmed. These responses show how animal control measures must be sensitive to the opinions of residents and tourists alike.

There seems no obvious way to characterize the group of tourists disenchanted by seeing roaming dogs. This may demonstrate the diversity of opinion concerning animal welfare. Responses of the tourists who were members of People for the Ethical Treatment of Animals were not in keeping with the sentiments expressed on the People for the Ethical Treatment of Animals website, which again shows the difficulty in trying to identify who may react negatively to seeing roaming dogs.

Twenty-eight percent of tourists were concerned about getting sick from the roaming dogs, whether or not they even saw the dogs, compared to the 65% of Bahamians who consider roaming dogs a health hazard "in general" (Table 8.2)—even though 5% of the tourists incorrectly thought The Bahamas has rabies. However, only 2% of all tourists felt scared or threatened by the dogs, and 5% of all Bahamians considered them a personal health hazard.

However, irrespective of any concerns about roaming dogs, 97% of the visitors enjoyed their stay and would either return or encourage others to visit. This reinforces the reactions given in Tables 9.2 and 9.3, that most tourists are insufficiently affected by the dogs, even if they did not like seeing roaming dogs, to discourage others to visit or themselves to visit again. With each visitor sharing their experiences with 15 others (and 2,000 in the case of a campus DJ), one disappointed tourist can have a disproportionate effect on a country's image and ultimately income. (It is worth remembering that even one percent of four million tourists is a large number of people, and their potential loss as tourists represents an important financial loss.) This explains the sensitivity of countries to foreign animal rights groups that post adverse comments on their Internet sites.[25] While such comments may be based on incidents of what welfare groups perceive to be poor animal welfare, the groups would do well to avoid distorting such reports as if they are the norm.

Overall, although relatively few tourists were upset to any degree by roaming dogs, it is possible for this minority to generate substantial adverse publicity about the country. In terms of tourist numbers, about 3,000 visitors per year may be distressed by the dogs, and they may deter as many as 42,000 other potential tourists from visiting. However, while considering the percentage of people offended by roaming dogs, it should be noted that far more, 6%, complain about litter,[26] and that there are other animals, such as pigs, which can attack tourists.[27] However, the potential lost revenue which can be attributed to roaming dogs indicates that it would be cost-effective for countries such as The Bahamas, which are dependent upon tourism for their livelihood, to invest large sums in controlling the dog population. Consequently, it is in the interest of both the dogs and country that animals are cared for.

10

Owned Dogs

[E]ven in upscale residential areas, pet dogs roam the streets at night. . . . Dogs, which have owners, should be confined to the owner's premises. Whether they are kept in the home at night or in the yard outside, they should be prevented access to the public road, unless they are with a person on a lead.[1]

Discussion of "owned" dogs is complicated by the fact that ownership is legally established by licensing an animal, which rarely happens, and the law also confers ownership of dogs when dogs spend most of their time on a person's property:

> "owner" shall include any person on whose premises a dog is found or whose premises a dog is known to frequent, unless such person can show that the dog is not his dog, and was on his premises without his consent.[2]

Thus, people legally own dogs which they might not consider as theirs, and others may claim to own dogs yet break the law by not licensing them. Many people do not understand these legal aspects of ownership; for example, some owners who keep their dogs confined do not think that it is necessary to license them; from our interviews and experiences it is clear that the wealthier as well as the poorer owners share this view.

Licensing of animals, although required by law,[3] has not been widespread, partly because until recently licenses were only available at one location, The Treasury. Relatively few dog licenses are distributed in relation to the size of the dog population, so even if all owners wished to license their animals, there would be a shortage of the license tag that a dog must wear.[4] Recently, veterinary clinics and post offices have started to sell dog licenses. We do not yet know if this change has resulted in a greater proportion of owned dogs being licensed. The license fees are $2 for a male or spayed female and $6 for an intact female.[5] The fine for owning an unlicensed dog is $40.[6] (As noted in Chapter 2, these fees are at historically low levels.) Thus, licensed dogs are a subset of owned dogs, with owners who are willing and able to license their animals; but we must remember that some owners willing to license their dogs are unable to do so. Bearing this in mind, we do not accept that 23% (of 142 replies) of the owners in our perception study had current licenses for their dogs,[7] yet this may, in some cases, reflect a genuine ignorance of the requirement for annual license renewal. Long-term observation of a street in an inner-city area found that 96% of the roaming dogs had no collars,[8] indicating that few dogs were formally owned (via licensing) by those people in contact with them. However, many of these dogs would have had a legal owner, as they were repeatedly seen in the same driveway or lying under the same car. This also indicates the difficulty which the authorities can have in establishing ownership should the need arise.

In order to simplify the matter, and put ownership in a context understood by residents, we consider owned dogs to be those that people claim to own, irrespective of legal technicalities. Thus, licensed dogs are considered a subgroup of owned dogs.

We use the term "breed" dog in accordance with local usage in New Providence rather than as a technical term. Therefore, "breed" may refer to a pure-bred (pedigree) dog (registered or unregistered) or to a dog which, although technically a cross, has a strong resemblance to a pure-bred dog. The term "cross-bred" is also now used to show that the animal has "some breed in him," rather than being "just" a potcake. In the strict use of the word, we feel, together with the Bahamas Humane Society, that there are very few pure-bred animals on the island, and that most are mixed. During the period 1982–2001, the Bahamas Kennel Club registered 911 pure-bred animals.[9] The list of the dogs registered by the Club is given in Table 10.1. The Club also registers litters, the most popular being Labradors, dachshunds, Dobermans and Pomeranians,[10] so the number of total canine registrations would be higher than that given in Table 10.1. If the figures are assumed to be indicators of the actual composition of pure-bred population, it can be seen that during 1982–1997, Dobermans, German shepherds and rottweilers accounted for 22% of registrations, while during 1998–2001 they accounted for 32%. As these breeds have increased in popularity, Labrador retrievers have become less fashionable, accounting for 13% of registration during 1982–1997 but only 8% in 1998–2001. These changes in the pattern of registrations may reflect an increasing use of these breeds for household security.[11]

Table 10.1: A list of dog breeds, and their numbers, registered by the Bahamas Kennel Club, 1982–2001.

Breed	1982–1997	1998–2001	Total
Labrador retriever	106	11	117
Doberman pinscher	54	30	84
German shepherd	64	3	67
Rottweiler	56	9	65
Dachshund	37	4	41
Poodle (standard & mini)	38	1	39
Golden retriever	26	1	27
American cocker spaniel	25	1	26
Boxer	22	3	25
Dalmatian	20	2	22
Shetland sheepdog	16	4	20

Breed	1982–1997	1998–2001	Total
Schnauzer (mini)	18	2	20
Belgian malinois	16	3	19
Chow-chow	16	2	18
Pomeranian	8	8	16
Yorkshire terrier	13	1	14
Great Dane	12	1	13
Collie	13		13
Fox terrier	13		13
Akita	10	2	12
English cocker spaniel	12		12
Siberian husky	12		12
Chihuahua	6	5	11
Poodle, toy	8	3	11
Shih tzu	9	2	11
Papillion	11		11
Jack Russell terrier*	6	4	10
Irish setter	10		10
Bulldog	8	1	9
Pug	9		9
Bull terrier	6	1	7
Maltese	6	1	7
Airedale terrier	7		7
Beagle	7		7
Bouvier des Flanders	7		7
Basset hound	5	1	6
German short haired pointer	5	1	6
Lhasa apso	6		6
Bedlington terrier	4	1	5
Bichon Frise	5		5
Samryed	5		5
Rhodesia ridgeback	3	1	4
Afghan hound	4		4
Saluki	4		4
Border collie		3	3
St. Bernard	1	2	3
Portuguese water dog	2	1	3
American Eskimo	3		3
Gordon setter	3		3
Mastiff	3		3
Pekingese	3		3
Chesapeake Bay retriever	1	1	2
American Staffordshire terrier	2		2
Australian terrier	2		2
Bull mastiff	2		2
Cairn terrier	2		2
English springer spaniel	2		2
Grey hound	2		2
Italian Greyhound	2		2
Keeshond	2		2
Pembroke Welsh corgi	2		2
Petit basset griffon Vendeen	2		2
Scottish terrier	2		2
Silky terrier	2		2

Breed	1982–1997	1998–2001	Total
Vizsla	2		2
Weimaraner	2		2
Japanese chin	1		1
Neapolitan mastiff	1		1
Toy fox terrier	1		1
TOTAL	780	131	911

* Jack Russells have only recently been recognized by the Club. Prior to this, owners had their own club.

The owned dog population is also augmented by imported dogs. The majority of dogs that come into the country (about 85%) belong to owners who are temporary residents or "tourists," and so they should not become part of the resident population.[12] A list of dogs imported into The Bahamas by owners with Bahamian addresses, in selected periods of 1997, 2000 and 2002 (Table 10.2), shows the range of breeds[13] entering the country and probably remaining here. Ninety percent of these dogs come from the United States.[14]

Table 10.2: A list of dog breeds, and their numbers, imported into The Bahamas in parts of 1997, 2000 and 2002 by residents.

Breed	1997	2000	2002	Total
Unspecified "mixed breed"	18	30	20	68
German shepherd (mix)	17 (2)	24 (2)	10 (2)	51 (6)
Rottweiler (mix)	23 (1)	19 (3)	3	45 (4)
Shih tzu	11	13	6	30
Yorkshire terrier	7	14	6	27
Labrador (mix)	6 (1)	15	1	22 (1)
Staffordshire terrier*[1]	5	9	7	21
Pomeranian	9	5	4	18
Chihuahua	6	8	3	17
Golden retriever	8	5	3	16
Boxer	9	4	2	15
Schnauzer	6	8	1	15
Poodle (mix)	8 (7)	4	1	13 (7)
Lhasa apso (mix)	6	7 (1)		13 (1)
Dachshund	7	4	2	13
American bull dog (mix)*	6	5 (2)	1	12 (2)
Jack Russell terrier	8	4		12
Chow-chow (mix)	7	3 (1)	1	11 (1)
Cocker spaniel	3	6	1	10
Pug	3	4	1	10
American Staffordshire terrier	1	6	2	9
Poodle, toy		8		8
Schnauzer (mini)	1	4	2	7
West Highland terrier[2]	5	1	1	7
Bichon Frise	3	2	1	6
Doberman pinscher	1	3	2	6
(Belgian?) Malinois	3	1		4
Toy dogs (mixed)		(4)		(4)
(Welsh?) Corgi	1	2		3
Akita[R]	3			3
Boston terrier		3		3
Bull mastiff			3	3

Bulldog	1	2		3
Coonhound[3]	2		1	3
King Charles spaniel		3		3
Maltese	1	2		3
Terrier, unspecified	1	2		3
Samryed (mix)	1 (1)	1		2 (1)
American terrier*[4]		2		2
Basset hound	2			2
Beagle	1	1		2
Bordeaux*		1	1	2
Collie		2		2
Dalmatian	2			2
Doberman pincher (min.)	2			2
Great Dane[R]		1	1	2
Mastiff		1	1	2
North American Spitz[5]	2			2
Pekingese	1	1		2
Shetland sheepdog	1	1		2
Airedale terrier	1			1
Alaskan malamute	1			1
American Eskimo	1			1
Australian Queensland*[6]			1	1
Australian shepherd	1			1
Basenji		1		1
Bull terrier		1		1
Chesapeake Bay retriever	1			1
Chinese Shar-Pei	1			1
Dachshund (mini)			1	1
Fox terrier				1
German short haired pointer[7]			1	1
Grey hound		1		1
Irish setter				1
Japanese spitz*	1			1
Old English sheep dog			1	1
Poodle (mini.)	1			1
Rhodesia ridgeback		1		1
Tibetan spaniel (mix)			1	1
Tibetan terrier	1			1
Weimaraner		1		1
Pomoek[8] (mix)		(1)		(1)
Dog, unspecified	1			1
TOTAL				588

* Not recognised by the American Kennel Club.   [R] = Observed to roam; see note 71.
1. The American Kennel Club recognises the American Staffordshire terrier and Staffordshire bull terrier. www.akc.org/breeds
2. Probably Scottish terriers.
3. Probably a black and tan Coonhound. One of these animals was reported lost and a $2,000 reward was offered. The Tribune (2002). Advertisement. 16 August, page 3.
4. Could be an American Staffordshire terrier.
5. Presumably related to the Finnish Spitz.
6. Might be an Australian shepherd.
7. Presumably a German wirehaired pointer.
8. Maybe a mistyping of Pomeranian.
Periods include April–September 1997; January–May 2000; and January–April 2002.
Numbers in parentheses refer to dogs of a stated mixed breed.

It is probably noteworthy that German shepherds are highly placed in both lists, and the observation is consistent with the idea of people owning dogs for protection. The most commonly advertised type of dog is the pit bull (30% of advertisements) and with a mean cost of $396 (se=$26.4).[15] The most commonly advertised breed is the Chow-chow (11% of advertisements) with a mean cost of $350 (se=$36.8).[16] The difference between the types of dogs advertised in the press and the dogs imported or registered may reflect the scale and scope of dogs bred for sale.

Results from the resident perception study

In December 1999, we interviewed 306 people in public places in New Providence in a convenience sample of adults. This study attempted to collect information on the extent of dog ownership and people's attitude and actions towards dogs. The results of the perception study (Table 10.3) outline many features of dog ownership in New Providence to which we shall refer to below. Other similar studies were also made in Abaco and produced similar results.[17] Therefore, in some instances we have used results from both islands to give a wider picture of ownership.

Table 10.3: Some aspects of dog ownership obtained from 306 interviews in New Providence.

Responses	%	Number responses
Own dogs	47	305
Keep dogs as pets/family animals	69	141
Keep dogs for protection	54	141
Take cat or dog to the veterinarian each year	34	164
Never take cat or dogs to the veterinarian	23	164
Keep dogs in a fenced-in yard	64	139
Allow their dogs to roam	28	141
Have at least one dog neutered	35	143
Abandon unwanted animals	9	45
Have disposed of animals at local humane groups	33	45
Have given away unwanted animals	29	45
Would use a humane society to dispose of unwanted animals	67	302
Consider local humane societies less than "effective"	57	300
Want more education on pet care for their children	98	300

Edited, revised and reproduced with permission from Fielding, W. J. and Mather, J. (2000). *Journal of Applied Animal Welfare Science* 3(4): 305–319. Not all questionnaires were fully completed. Some questions were only asked to the relevant subpopulation of interviewees.

From Table 10.3 it can be appreciated that many people keep dogs for security and as "pets," but relatively few owners take their dogs to the veterinarian regularly. While many dogs are kept in a fenced yard, many do roam, and if the fence is not stock-proof, many more animals may have access to the road than owners think (see Chapter 7). Nearly 40% of owners have disposed of or abandoned unwanted animals, and this is associated with a low percentage of owners having at least one animal neutered. Although most people said they would dispose of excess dogs humanely, about 10% admitted to abandoning animals. As abandonment is a sensitive issue, this figure may underestimate the actual value. Almost all our interviewees wanted more education for children on pet issues, and this may reflect their own lack of education on pet welfare (see Chapter 7).

Table 10.4: Mean numbers of owned dogs, by age and class of owner, in New Providence.

	Under 35 years		
	Sole male	Sole female	Joint
Male dogs	1.16 (se=0.122)	0.97 (se=0.193)	1.48 (se=0.197)
Neutered males	0.22 (se=0.059)	0.12 (se=0.055)	0.50 (se=0.129)
Female dogs	0.96 (se=0.140)	1.00 (se=0.224)	1.10 (se=0.215)
Neutered females	0.22 (se=0.066)	0.15 (se=0.061)	0.62 (se=0.187)
All dogs	2.10 (se=0.186)	1.97 (se=0.373)	2.57 (se=0.343)
All neutered dogs	0.44 (se=0.091)	0.26 (se=0.076)	1.15 (se=0.288)
No. of values	50	35	42
	35 years or over		
	Sole male	Sole female	Joint
Male dogs	1.48 (se=0.168)	1.23 (se=0.244)	1.40 (se=0.183)
Neutered males	0.67 (se=0.166)	0.40 (se=0.141)	0.60 (se=0.167)
Female dogs	1.10 (se=0.189)	1.00 (se=0.151)	1.37 (se=0.157)
Neutered females	0.62 (se=0.187)	0.68 (se=0.154)	0.97 (se=0.165)
All dogs	2.57 (se=0.288)	2.23 (se=0.273)	2.77 (se=0.269)
All neutered dogs	1.29 (se=0.294)	1.02 (se=0.214)	1.57 (se=0.282)
No. of values	42	44	63

Extent of ownership

Overall, in New Providence, respondents owned an average of 1.23 (se=0.119) dogs, and there were 2.60 (se=0.20) dogs per dog-owning household. A relatively small number of people own most of the dogs. When the data from the perception studies in New Providence and Abaco[18] are combined, the Lorenz curve in Figure 10.1 is obtained.[19] In another study,[20] we found that owners had a mean of 2.44 (se=0.120) dogs, 39% of owners had only one dog, and older owners (those over 35 years old) had more dogs than younger owners (p<0.001) (Table 10.4). Similar patterns of ownership have been seen elsewhere, for example, Sri Lanka.[21]

Our subsequent studies have suggested that less than 45% of households own dogs, so the curve maybe even more extreme than shown in Figure 10.1. In our health study (described in Chapter 15) 32% of patients lived in dog-owning households. In Bain Town and Yamacraw, 48% and 60% (each of 35 respondents) of households owned dogs.[22] From the replies of respondents contacted by telephone in our neuter study (discussed in Chapter 12), we could conclude that 21% of households have dogs.

But it should be noted that since "ownership" is often a personal issue, the respondent may not "own" dogs even though there may be dogs in the household, and telephone surveys find lower levels of pet ownership than in face-to-face interviews.[23]

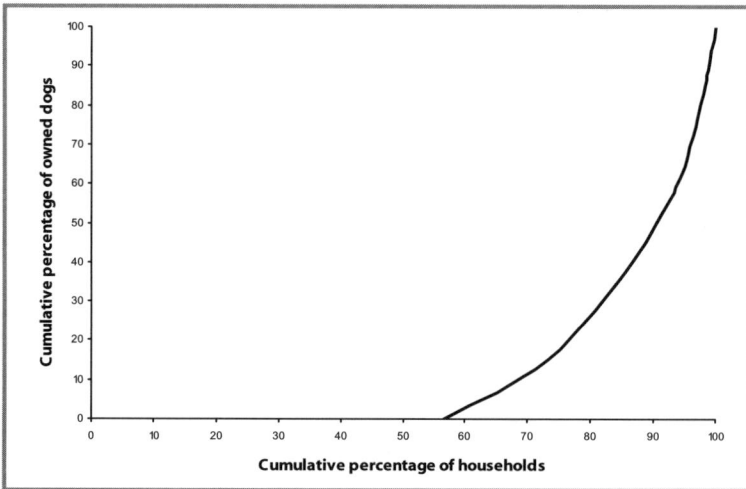

Figure 10.1: Lorenz curve of the distribution of dog ownership (of 448 dogs) across 410 households in The Bahamas.
Reproduced with permission from Fielding, W. J. and Mather, J. (2001). Dog ownership in the West Indies: A case study from The Bahamas. *Anthrozoös* 14(2): 72–80.

These figures put limits on the extent of dog ownership. Thus, the extent of claimed ownership is less than elsewhere, e.g., 68% of households in Costa Rica, 64% in Australia, and 58–59% in the US.[24] Figure 10.1 shows that the common complaint that New Providence suffers from a "stray dog problem" is probably caused by a minority of the population, and that relatively few owners (10%) own the majority of the dogs (50%).

Reasons for ownership

The most common reason for owning a dog was as a family "pet." This response must be viewed in the light of our discussion in Chapter 5. Thus it would seem that "as a pet" should be considered to mean an animal that is cared for, rather than a companionable animal, for most of the 69% of the owners in the study who have dogs as pets. In fact, 28% of owners said that they kept the dogs as a pet and for protection, so at most 41% of owners kept their dogs only "as a pet." Elsewhere, for example in Ecuador, an even greater percentage of owners keep dogs for protection.[25] The fact that 54% of owners said the dogs were for "protection" emphasizes the protective aspects of pets and dogs. Some residents even give the use of dogs for protection as a reason why owners allow their dogs to roam,[26] which may be an attempt to protect the street as much as a particular property. However, if people use a dog to protect their home, the police advise the use of a small dog which can be kept inside.[27] It should be remembered that probably most of the dogs kept to protect homes are potcakes. Interestingly, a student in one of our studies considered potcakes as "inferior" guard dogs, an observation in agreement with data from our study on dogs and security. Another student stated that "they don't do anything, but they do bark," thus suggesting that potcakes are used as "burglar alarms," that is, they are used as watch dogs. However, others consider them to be excellent guard dogs.[28] "Image" dogs, such as rottweilers, are also used to guard homes, even in poorer communities of Nassau.[29] Table 5.3 indicated the importance of selected reasons why neighbours were thought to keep dogs. It is clear that companionable aspects of dog ownership are thought to be secondary to protection.

Composition of the owned dog population

More male (59%) than female dogs (41%) were licensed (p<0.05), and this preference was shown irrespective of the type of dog (p=0.4). In the more general population of owned dogs (i.e., dogs which are probably unlicensed), over half (53%) of the population was composed of males (361 of 678),[30] which again shows a preference for male dogs (p=0.04). No preference for dogs of a particular sex by any particular class of owner could be found. Sole male, sole female and joint owners had a similar number of male dogs (1.30, s.e.=0.076) (p=0.14), and these classes of owners also had similar numbers of female dogs (1.14, s.e.=0.80) (p=0.40).[31]

As indicated above, we know that most of the dogs in New Providence are potcakes, but a wide range of pure-bred animals are also imported. In Abaco, the Labrador is the most commonly imported pure-bred dog, and there about 75% of owned dogs were estimated to be potcakes.[32] Results from a small-scale study[33] that looked at the relative abundance of different types of dog within the general owned population found that 68% (of 62 dogs) were potcakes. Another small-scale study of 41 owners found that 7% owned pit bulls, 5% German shepherds and the remainder, 88%, owned potcakes/mixed breeds.[34] However, our daily observations suggest that these may still be underestimates of the proportion of potcakes.

The Bahamas Kennel Club registers an average of about 46 dogs a year, and we estimate that about 1,100 pure-bred dogs are imported a year, so we could expect pure-bred dogs to make up about 10% of the owned dog population. If only 15% of imported dogs actually remain here, then pure-bred dogs may make up about 2% of the resident owned dog population.

In New Providence, the Bahamas Kennel Club has indicated that rottweilers and rottweiler mixes have been popular in recent years. Their popularity is reflected in the relatively high numbers of rottweilers imported (Table 10.2) and their position in Table 10.5. Not surprisingly, given the links between America and The Bahamas, the more common breeds imported into New Providence are reflected in the ranking of breeds registered with the American Kennel Club in recent years.[35] Of the four most commonly registered breeds by the Bahamas Kennel Club, three could be considered as guard breeds. Similarly, the top two breeds imported into The Bahamas are German shepherds and rottweilers. Such figures seem to confirm the demand for dogs to provide protection.

Reflecting the preferences in America and elsewhere of "image" dogs, pit bulls first started being noticeable in 1980s,[36] and they have been reported as being the most popular type on the island. Data from two veterinary clinics show that after potcakes, pit bulls were the most common dogs seen,[37] followed by rottweilers. These observations confirm claims made in the press and indicate that residents favour dogs with histories of biting behaviour.[38] The consequences of this preference are discussed further in Chapter 16.

Table 10.5: Composition of adult dogs, by type, seen at two veterinary clinics in New Providence in 2001.

Type	Percentage
Potcake	31
Pit bull	28
Rottweiler	18
German shepherd	5
Labrador	2
Spaniel	1
Others	16

For reasons of confidentiality the actual number of dogs is not given, but exceeds 5,000.

While Table 10.5 gives a ranking of the relative numbers of some types of dogs, the percentage of potcakes given in the table is certainly an underestimate of the importance of potcakes in the general population, because many potcakes never visit the veterinarian.[39]

Age structure of owned dogs

We consider age to be an important indicator of animal welfare, although we are aware of its limitations.[40] Therefore, we shall consider age from several aspects in our description of owned dogs.

Data on the ages of owned dogs were available from a convenience sample study[41] and from dog license records. These two sources of data were combined in order to get a larger picture of the age structure of the owned dog population (Figure 10.2). This age distribution is consistent with the hypothesis that 27% of the population dies each year (p>0.05). We regard this age structure as being primarily that of a potcake population, as potcakes are the most common type of dog.

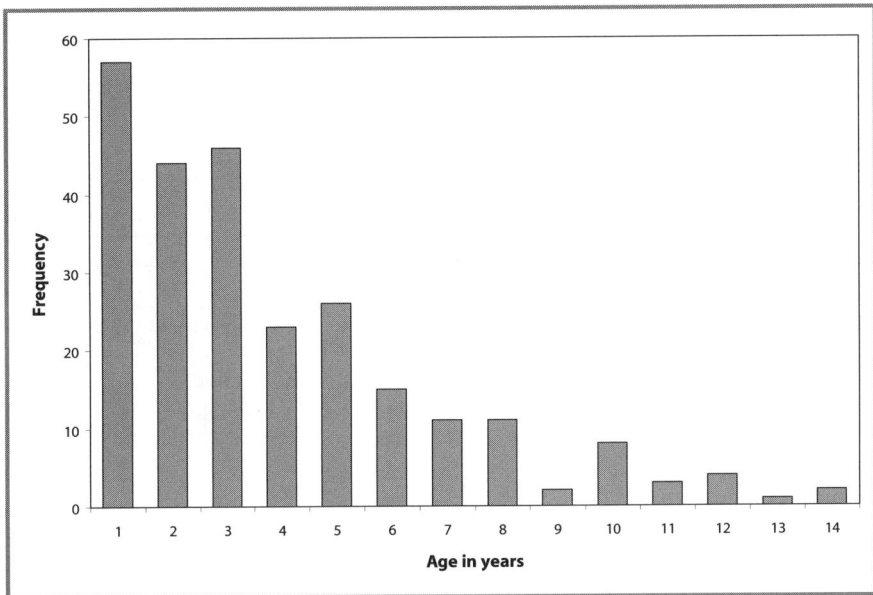

Figure 10.2: Distribution of the ages of 337 dogs (owned or licensed) in The Bahamas.
Reproduced from Fielding, W. J. and Mather, J. (2001) with permission. Dog ownership in the West Indies: A case study from The Bahamas. *Anthrozoös* 14(2): 72–80.

Only 12% of the population is over seven years of age and the median age is three years. This age structure is similar to that found in Barbados, Ecuador, Sri Lanka and Tunisia,[42] but it also indicates that owned dogs live less long in The Bahamas than more northerly territories. For example, in the US state of Indiana, the median age is five years, and 30% are over seven years old.[43] Other studies have estimated the median life expectancy for cross-bred dogs as thirteen years and seven years for some pure-breeds.[44]

From the dog license records we can get further details regarding ages and types of dog and their breeding status. When licensed and merely "owned" dogs are separated, they are found to have similar age structures, as seen in Table 10.6. Although males and females have the same median age, more females live over six years than males (Table 10.7).

The term "cross-bred" was used by some owners to distinguish between a mixed-bred animal which still shows clear traits of a recognized breed, and a potcake, which has no obvious traits of any breed. We have differentiated cross-bred from potcake to reflect this owner-based classification. When ages of licensed dogs are compared by type of dog—potcake, mixed (or cross) bred or pure-bred—little difference is found between the ages of the three types (Table 10.8). A possible explanation for this similarity in average age of all types of dogs may be the effect of heartworm and adequate access to veterinary care on the population.

Table 10.6: A summary of the ages (years) of two classes of dogs in The Bahamas.

	Licensed dogs	"Owned" dogs
25 percentile	1.5	1.75
50 percentile (median)	3.0	3.0
75 percentile	5.0	4.25
Sample size	256	84

Owned dogs: These are claimed to be owned, but are probably, but not necessarily, unlicensed.

Table 10.7: Percentile points of the ages (in years) of male and female dogs licensed in 1999.

	Males	Females
25 percentile	1	2
50 percentile	3	3
75 percentile	5	6

Table 10.8: Percentile points of the ages (in years) of three classes of licensed dogs.

	Potcake	Cross-breed	Pure-breed
25 percentile	1.9	1.0	1.1
50 percentile	3.0	3.0	3.0
75 percentile	5.0	6.0	6.0

Effect of neutering on dog age

Neutered dogs have a higher average age than intact animals (Table 10.9). This observation probably arises from the fact that intact dogs may suffer from sexually transmitted diseases,[45] stress associated with mating, fighting and exposure to other diseased dogs; additionally, in the case of females, they may be weakened as a result of poor health care and over-breeding.

Amongst the licensed dog population, pure-bred dogs are the least likely and potcakes the most likely to be neutered (Table 10.10). These actions are in line with the fact that potcakes are considered as worthless animals (they are not sold, even by a pet shop), whereas pure-bred animals can fetch many hundreds of dollars. Pit bull puppies can fetch $700,[46] which indicates the demand for such animals. Of the 19 licensed pit bulls ("pure" or cross-bred), only 26% were neutered, which is less than the 62% (p<0.01) of all other types of dog. This observation might be a consequence of a government policy of not granting import licenses for pit bulls.[47] It should also be remembered that pit bulls are the most common breed type seen at veterinary clinics. This observation is consistent with the finding in our neuter study, where the most common reason given for not neutering dogs was because people wanted to breed them.

Table 10.9: Percentile points of the ages (in years) of neutered and intact dogs licensed in 1999.

	Neutered	Intact
25 percentile	2	1
50 percentile	3	2
75 percentile	6	4

Table 10.10: Percentage of licensed dogs classified by breed and breeding status.

	Neutered	Intact
Pure-bred (n=81)	51	49
Potcake (n=134)	64	36
Cross-bred (n=38)	55	45

Licensed females are more likely to be neutered (72%) than males (51%) (p<0.001). In a more general population, neuter rates were lower: 50% percent of females (of 318 dogs) and 34% of males (of 361 animals). This again confirms the higher neuter rate of female dogs.[48]

Effect of habitat on dog age[49]

Most owners keep their dogs outside the house, usually in order to protect the household. Once the dogs are outside the house, it becomes easy for them to wander and interact with other roaming dogs and be put at risk of harm from cars,[50] people and other dogs. From Table 10.11 it can be seen that either keeping dogs outside the home or allowing them to roam negatively affects their welfare, as fewer such dogs live beyond four years of age, compared to confined dogs. Dogs that are confined have a higher average age than those which are not (p<0.01), and dogs kept inside the home have a higher average age than those which are not (p<0.05).

Dogs that are both confined and kept inside the home have the highest median age (six years). The mean age of those animals always kept inside the house is higher than that of any other group (p<0.05); see Table 10.12.

Table 10.11: Ages (years) of owned dogs classified by place of habitation and ability to roam.

	25%ile	50%ile	75%ile	N
Dogs confined	2	4	6	40
Dogs kept inside the house	2	3	10	21
Dogs kept outside the house	1.5	3	4	63
Dogs allowed to roam	1	3	3	45

Table 10.12: Median ages (years) of owned dogs classified by place of habitation and ability to roam.

	Allowed to roam	Confined
Kept inside the house	2	6
Kept outside the house	3	4

Effect of visiting the veterinarian[51]

About 25% of owners never take their dogs to the veterinarian (Table 10.3).[52] It would seem logical that animals that visit the veterinarian belong to owners who are more aware of the health needs of their animals. The result of the owner's contact with a veterinarian should result in a more informed owner, and thus the welfare of the animal should be improved. We are aware, however, that many owners may only bring puppies to the clinic for their vaccinations, and so visits to the clinic may not necessarily be associated with a group of animals with a higher average age. Therefore, we have attempted to look at other indicators that which might be associated with level of animal care.

Statistically, no differences in the ages of animals and frequency of visiting a clinic could be found. However, we feel that this lack of association is due to our small sample size rather than anything else, as the data in Table 10.13 suggest that visiting the clinic, no matter how often, is better for the dog (as measured by average age) than no visit at all.

Table 10.13: A summary of the ages (years) of owned dogs by frequency of visits to a veterinarian.

	No visit	When necessary	At least once a year
25 percentile	1	2	2
50 percentile	2	4	3
75 percentile	4	5	4
Sample size	13	34	40

As would be expected, very few animals which never visit a clinic are neutered.[53] Presumably these are dogs which have been given away or adopted after being neutered, and the present owners have never taken the animal back to the veterinarian (Table 10.14).

Table 10.14: Percentages of owners with neutered dogs classified by frequency to veterinary clinics.

	Annually	When needed	Never
Unneutered	54	58	94
Neutered	46	42	6
No. of replies	52	59	33

Figures also include visits to clinics for cats, but few cats were reported in the New Providence perception study.

The habitat of the dog provides an indicator as to whether or not the animal visits the veterinarian. Almost a third of all owners who kept their animals outside the house had never taken them to the clinic, compared with only 13% of dog owners keeping their animals inside the house (Table 10.15). Of those owners who never take their animals to the clinic, 13% kept their dogs inside the house and 87% kept them outside the house, but the sample size is too small to indicate a statistically significant difference.[54] Our larger study, in New Providence, which only classified habitat as a fenced or unfenced yard, found that 16% of the owners who kept their animals in a fenced yard never took their animals to the clinic, compared with 47% who did not keep their animals in a fenced yard (p<0.001).[55]

Table 10.15: Percentage of owners in Abaco keeping their dogs in selected places by frequency of visit to veterinarians.

	Once a year	When necessary	Never	n
Kept inside the house	63	25	13	8
Kept outside the house	40	32	28	25

Health care of the owned potcake

Potcakes have less access to health care than pure-bred dogs. In one veterinary clinic in Abaco, as few as 10% of the dogs taken to the clinic were potcakes, although potcakes made up 75% or more of the dog population.[56] This observation was in broad agreement in New Providence, where potcakes only made up 30% of the dogs seen in two private veterinary clinics (Table 10.5). Ensuring that dogs are kept healthy at an early age has shown to reduce a number of problematical behaviours later on.[57] These include barking, aggression towards strangers and fear of strangers, three behaviours often associated with potcakes. Possibly, better health care early on could lessen some of the problematical behaviours which potcakes can exhibit.

The potcake has a reputation of being a "survivor" and therefore in need of little attention.[58] Our observations appear to support this view, because potcakes, while receiving less medical attention than pure-bred animals, have a similar average age. Thus despite their lack of health care, they live just as long as pure-bred dogs. However, we know of potcakes which received good health care and lived to 12 years or more.

Fecundity of owned dogs[59]

In the 12 months prior to our study 31 owned females had produced 24 puppies. This is an average pup/mother survival rate of 0.77 puppies/female. Some mothers had been spayed after giving birth, so the number of surviving puppies per litter was 3.4. As all these females had been allowed to roam, it is possible that none of these litters were planned, and that most, if not all, the puppies were surplus to the owners' needs.[60] Such unintentional litters result in puppies that are most likely to be abandoned.[61] If they are abandoned, owners are transferring owned dogs to the free-roaming, unowned population. The importance of this transfer is discussed in connection with our "balance sheet" (Table 10.16).

Dog ownership in minority groups

It is recognized that minority groups may look after their dogs differently from the general population which we have studied. For example, we have not attempted to investigate how the Haitian community (the largest non-national group in The Bahamas[62]) cares for its dogs. We feel that such a study might highlight interesting differences in the way Bahamians and Haitians look after their pets due to the nature of their settlements,[63] background and their economic resources.

Attitudes towards welfare groups

Many people feel dissatisfied with the local humane societies.[64] This dissatisfaction should be considered when noting that 67% of our respondents claimed that they would take unwanted animals to the shelter. However, there is a perception that surrendering animals is a death sentence (as described in Stubbs' song; see page 19) and this may encourage active abandonment in the pine barrens or other sparsely populated areas.[65] However, it should be noted than many people still do surrender unwanted animals to humane groups (Table 10.3). Resistance to surrendering was illustrated by a neighbour accusing WF of being "a murderer" when he called the Animal Control Unit to remove puppies, born to an owned, roaming dog, which were hiding under his neighbours' cars.[66]

Owned roaming dogs

Although only 28% of owners claimed to let their dogs roam, we feel this is an underestimate. In the strict interpretation of the word "roam," we feel that the number is closer to 40%. In our neuter study, 42% of dogs were allowed to roam and in Abaco 50% of the dogs were allowed to roam.[67] However, most respondents would interpret the question as "roam often" rather than at all,[68] so in this respect 28% may not be such a gross underestimate. However, when considering breeding opportunities we believe that a strict interpretation is required, so it is clear that a large section of the owned dog population probably has the opportunity to breed at will.[69] The law is also strict on forbidding dogs "in heat" to roam and the fine is $100.[70] Although most of the dogs which roam are potcakes, pure-bred dogs are also allowed to roam.[71]

Despite the high percentage of owners who let their dogs roam, Bahamian dog owners are not alone in letting their dogs roam. In Sri Lanka, only 27% of dogs are never allowed to roam and 34% roam all the time. In Tunisia, about 30% of dogs always roam and in Ecuador 29% of dogs roam.[72]

A current neutering programme has now focussed its neutering efforts only on owned dogs. This is because owned dogs are expected to have better nutrition than roaming dogs and so a greater breeding potential. Given the large number of owned dogs which roam, this strategy could reduce the number of puppies which find their way into the unowned population.

Reasons for allowing owned dogs to roam[73]

Seventy-one percent of residents agreed that the most common reason for dogs roaming was because they were not fed by the owner.[74] This perception is consistent with the admission by 53% of dog owners (of 38 respondents)[75] that they did not feed their dogs each day. For some owners, allowing dogs to roam may be convenient, as owners would not need to clean up dog faeces or feed them regularly. The use of dogs for protection was considered by 40% of respondents in Bain Town but only 8% in Yamacraw (p=0.014) as a reason why dogs were allowed to roam. Presumably, owners think that a confined dog will be able to rush out and bark at an intruder. Although many residents thought that adult dogs could take care of themselves (49% of respondents in Bain Town and 74% in Yamacraw) and so it was acceptable to let the dogs roam, these responses indicate large local variations (p=0.05) on this issue, which might be location-related.

Thus the responses indicate that some dogs roam in search of food to supplement their diet, and that some residents think that dogs need to be mobile to protect a property. However, these reasons might suggest that people underestimate the real dangers dogs face from cars, theft, etc., when they are free to roam. As indicated in a hand-painted road sign, residents tend to blame car drivers for hitting dogs, not the owners for allowing the dogs to roam.

Interaction between owned and roaming dogs

The "balance sheet" (Table 10.16) below is based on information provided by our surveys and supplemented with data from other local sources. It aims to show the approximate gains and losses to the dog population in a year. Clearly, the actual numbers are less important than the relative sizes of the gains and losses. The assumptions and details of the estimates are given in Appendix 2.

The balance sheet shows that the owned and unowned populations are interconnected by the actions of owners and society in general. These linkages are important, as it can be seen that human behaviour can limit or increase the unowned dog population. The most obvious linkage is through abandonment.[76] If owners stopped abandoning animals (either actively by leaving animals in "remote" areas, such as the pine barrens[77] or passively by (for example) leaving their pets behind when they move[78]), the unowned population could be expected to decline. We should also remember that some animals reported "stolen" (see Table 13.1) could represent additional recruits to the unowned population as they may have wandered off as a result of neglect. "Lost" notices in the press could indicate that owned dogs might simply wander off from their homes.[79] Further, it can be seen that relatively few dogs may be imported each year.[80] The relatively large number of animals killed through human actions indicates the risk of dogs suffering a painful death, and the dangers to which roaming dogs are exposed. The conclusions from Table 10.16 concur with those found in other studies of dog populations and highlight the dependency of the roaming population on recruitment from the owned population for its survival.[81]

Table 10.16: An indicative balance sheet of the owned and unowned dog populations in New Providence, for the year starting January 2000.

	Owned	Balance	Unowned	Balance
Opening balance[1]	73,200	73,200	11,100	11,100
Deaths[2]	19,800	53,400	6,000	5,100
Imports[3]	325	53,725		
Abandoned/recruits[4]	7,200	46,425	7,200	12,300
Removed by ACU[5]	400	46,025	1,200	11,100
Poisoned[6]	600	45,425	1,400	9,700
Killed on roads[7]	600	44,825	1,600	8,100
Births[8]	29,175	74,000	3,100	11,200
Closing balance	74,000		11,200	

1. From our resident perception studies.
2. Based on Figure 10.2 for owned dogs and assuming twice the mortality for unowned dogs.
3. Anon (2000). Report for the month of January–December 1999. Department of Agriculture, The Bahamas. However, a subsequent investigation by us of 216 import permits issued in 2000 suggests that only 17% were issued to Bahamian residents, so in a 12-month period only 215 permits might be issued which result in permanent additions to the dog population. On average about 1.5 dogs are imported on each permit. Our estimate of the number imported is probably an underestimate because it does not include imports by pet shops.
4. From our perception study in New Providence.
5. Based on data presented about the Animal Control Unit above.
6. The Tribune (2000). Pets in danger from poisoners. 12 May, p. 4.
7. Hepburn, L. (2000). Personal communication. Department of Environmental Health, Nassau. However, deaths or injuries to dogs by motor vehicles are not recent, and go back to at least 1965. The Nassau Guardian (1965). Letter to the editor. 4 February, p. 6.
8. Inferred, so that closing balances are no more than 1% more than the opening balances. This limit ties the population growth with the number of new households per year estimated by the Department of Statistics, Nassau.

11

The Role of Dogs in Household Security

Are you worried about the crime situation in Nassau? Do you feel safe at work, going home, or walking to your car without protection? No? Well buy a dog now for your safety ...[1]

As has been seen earlier, security is a common, if not primary, reason for owning dogs. With so many people owning dogs for security, it is important to know if dogs do actually provide householders protection from criminals, and if not, why not. Also, what are the implications for the dogs (mainly potcakes) "employed" to protect homes?

A preliminary study on the effectiveness of dogs as a deterrent in protecting 229 homes (81% were houses or bungalows) of students at The College of The Bahamas found that a similar percentage of households were attacked (33%) irrespective of the presence or absence of dogs (p=0.77). Even when other security measures were considered (e.g., location of the home in relation to vacant lots etc., night security lights, security bars, etc.) the presence of dogs in the home did not reduce the chance of the home being attacked (p=0.30). Given that "a dog" did not appear to provide security, the data were further analyzed to try to find out why this might be.

Homes with dogs

Ninety-two percent of owners kept their dogs outside all the time (75 replies). While 61% of owners said that their dogs were kept in an area from which they could not escape, and 42% of households (of 74 replies) allowed their dogs to get onto the street. Fifty-four percent of owners (of 65 replies) kept their dogs in a locked stock-proof area and in 71% of the homes dogs had access to all sides of the property. Twenty-four percent of (148) dogs were said to be "attack-trained." How the owners kept the dogs was associated with the chances of homes being attacked (Table 11.1). From the results

97

in Table 11.1 it is apparent that confinement of the dogs is important in reducing the chances of attack on the home.

Table 11.1: A comparison of dog-owning homes which were broken into, classified by aspects of dog care.

Response to question:	%age broken into within each group		p
	Yes	No	
Dogs can get onto the street?	45	26	0.089
Dogs usually kept outside only?	33	33	1.00
Dogs have access to all sides of the home?	32	36	0.79
Dogs kept in a locked stock-proof area?	23	40	0.18
Dogs kept in an area from which they cannot escape?	20	55	0.002

Maximum number of responses, 75; 10 households with dogs did not respond.

When homes were attacked, 54% of respondents (24 replies) claimed that their dogs were on the property at the time of the attack and 42% did not know if they were. Similarly, 79% of respondents did not know if the dog had barked when the attack took place. When a home had been attacked, 33% of respondents reported that their dogs had been harmed either prior to or during the attack (24 replies).

Potcakes compared with breed dogs

Homes were classified as to whether or not they owned only potcakes ("only potcake" owning homes) and those which owned at least one purebred or a dog which looked like a purebred dog, even if it also owned potcakes ("homes with pure-breed dogs"). It was assumed that all the dogs belonging to a household were kept in the same way.

As we would expect, the most commonly reported types of dogs were potcakes. Fifty-five percent (of 155 dogs) were potcakes, 10% chow-chows, 9% pit bulls and 9% German shepherds.[2] However, we feel that many of the declared purebreds are probably cross-breeds, because, as we noted earlier, there are relatively few purebred dogs on the island. Overall, 38% percent of the dogs were neutered and 62% were males.[3]

Seven percent of potcakes were "attack-trained," compared to 50% of purebred dogs (137 dogs) (p<0.001). Eighty-three percent of "attack-trained" dogs were kept in an area from which they could not escape, compared with 60% of untrained dogs (141 dogs) (p<0.006). Forty-eight percent of potcakes could get onto the street, compared with 25% of purebred dogs (146 dogs) (p<0.001). All respondents from homes with "attack-trained" dogs thought that the dogs had been successful in protecting the home. Fifty-six percent (of 18 homes) with at least one "attack-trained" dog were in households which had children.

Simple inspection of the percentage of homes with and without a purebred dog showed that 49% of homes with only potcakes were attacked, compared with 17% of homes with at least one purebred dog (p=0.005) (73 homes). This result suggests that owning only potcakes provides a minimal deterrent to criminals. However, homes with at least one purebred kept their dogs differently from homes with only potcakes. Forty-five percent of homes with only potcakes kept them in an area from which they could not escape, compared with 74% of purebreds (p=0.02) (66 homes). In homes with only potcakes, 40% of the dogs were kept in a locked area, compared with 66% of homes with purebreds (p=0.067) (60 homes) (Table 11.2). A similar percentage of respondents from homes with and without only potcakes (80%) did not know if their dogs had barked during a successful attack (p=0.64) (20 homes).

Table 11.2: Aspects of dog care classified by type of dogs owned.

| Type of dog in the home | % of homes | | p |
	Potcakes only	At least one "purebred"	
Home attacked	48	17	<0.01
Dogs usually kept outside only	100	90	0.20
Dogs have access to all sides of the home	66	74	0.59
Dogs can get onto the street	50	36	0.32
Dogs kept in area from which they cannot escape	45	74	0.02
Dogs kept in a locked stock-proof area	40	66	0.07

Percentage of households within each class. (Maximum number of responses 73). Households with "purebreds" includes homes with at least one dog which looked like a purebred or included at least one pit bull.

Respondents from both homes with only potcakes or purebred dogs were in similar agreement (70%) that their dogs had been successful in protecting their homes (p=0.36) (67 homes). Likewise, a similar percentage of homes reported that their dogs were harmed either before or during an attack, whether they owned only potcakes or at least one breed dog (25%) (20 replies).

Eighty-two percent of (73 replies) of respondents in households which had not been attacked thought that dogs had been successful in protecting their homes, compared with 46% when households had been attacked (p=0.007). Respondents in homes with only potcakes were in similar agreement with respondents with purebreds that their dogs had been successful in protecting their home (p=0.36)

Comments

The observations that most households and most dogs are owned for protection are consistent with our other studies which found that protection was considered a more important reason for dog ownership than companionship. The pattern of ownership—having many dogs (usually intact), which are kept outside, and/or can roam—does not appear to be conducive to dogs' being effective protectors of the household. Complaints by residents about owners who allow "fierce" dogs to roam is consistent with this finding.[4] Further, when dogs are kept outside, they are at risk from being harmed either before or during an attack, possibly by being poisoned,[5] so being kept as a deterrent to criminals is not without risk to the dog, whether or not it is a potcake. Further, when dogs are kept outside they are at risk of themselves being stolen.[6]

Different breeds of dogs are attributed with different merits for home protection,[7] but the ability to consistently sound the alarm at intruders is less well associated with breed than other characteristics.[8] It would appear that in New Providence chow-chows, pit bulls and German shepherds are the current dogs of choice for protection, all dogs with noted biting behaviour.[9] Pit bulls are the most frequently advertised dogs for sale in the press, and they are the most common type seen by veterinarians in New Providence. They have been almost certainly responsible for all the fatalities due to dog attacks in the island, and the consequences of them being allowed to roam have been much discussed.[10] Due to the perceived danger these dogs pose to society, some groups have even wanted these animals banned.[11] Despite the popular perceptions about pit bulls, this study did not find them as the overwhelmingly common guard dog of choice.

Although many respondents claimed that their dogs were "attack-trained," we feel that this reflects the perception of the respondent, and the dogs are better considered as aggressive. The actual number of formally attack-trained dogs is probably less than reported here, as we know of few owners who have professionally trained dogs. However, having attack-trained or aggressive dogs in a household setting is not recommended, as they might injure household members.[12] The ability of attack-trained pit bulls to kill in a commercial setting has already been demonstrated in New Providence.[13] Over half of the homes reportedly having attack-trained dogs included children, which means that householders may be putting their own children and their children's friends at risk.[14]

The fact that so many owners did not know if their dogs barked or were on the property when the attack took place suggests that the owners were absent during the attack. This is consistent with the fact that most attacks on property take place during the day, when, presumably, the home is unoccupied.[15] Although the dogs may "bark a lot" when the owner is at home, the ability of the dog to effectively raise an alarm when the owner is absent may be less. Further, in areas where there are many barking dogs, the warning provided by a particular dog probably becomes less effective.

As indicated earlier, the common perception in New Providence is that dogs provide "protection" and are kept to protect homes; this perception was reiterated by dog owners in this study, particularly by owners whose homes had never been attacked. However, this study does not support the perception that a generic dog actually enhances the security of a household. Although this study gives the impression that potcakes do not make good guard dogs (and several respondents supported this view), it is not possible to say that "purebred" dogs are actually better, as they are more likely to be confined, and more likely to be "attack-trained" than potcakes. Thus, it is not clear if it is all the factors—confinement, training or breed—or a combination that influence a dog's ability to protect a home. The difference in care towards potcakes and "purebred" was also seen in our case studies.

Despite the preliminary nature of the study, just owning a dog can constitute little or no deterrent to a criminal, other than, maybe, to an opportunist. An example of this was reported in the press, when the presence of both potcake and purebred dogs failed to protect their owners from attack.[16] In most cases, this ineffectiveness is almost certainly increased by the fact that many owners do not confine their dogs. This finding disagrees with the attitudes of owners, and so suggests that it will be hard to change their beliefs. Not only does the way owners keep their dogs prevent the animals from fulfilling their purpose, but it also exposes them to danger. We feel that while changes in the way dogs are kept may help to enhance their deterrent effect, and also reduce the number of roaming dogs on the streets, householders should look to additional methods of deterring criminal attacks on their homes, particularly houses.

We note that since 1990 the percentage of residents in all The Bahamas living in single houses has decreased from 68%[17] to 62%[18] in 2000, while the percentage living in apartments and townhouses has increased from 13% to 17%. This change in type of accommodation might result in reduced dog ownership, as townhouses etc. tend to have more in-built security than a single house. (Additionally, townhouse complexes often forbid dog ownership.) This in turn should lessen the requirement for residents to own dogs for protection. If this happens, the importance of dog ownership for "security" should diminish, which should be beneficial to the dogs.

12

Attitudes and Actions towards Neutering

The dogs breed too fast—the island's population is too big.[1]

In a single newspaper 13 advertisements appeared for dogs: (1) Pitbulls "blue full-bread" and brindle, (2) "Full German bred" Rot Wilders,[2] (3) "Awesome chocolate red nose" pit bulls (4) "Beautiful Doberman," (5) "Black miniature poodles," (6) "Burn-side pitt bull read nose" puppies (7) "Champayne pittbull" puppies, (8) Chihuahua puppies (9) "Pitbull puppies" (10) Pitbull puppies (11) "Adorable Japanese Spitz," (12) "Rotwiler and Doberman mixed" (13) "White/blue & white/fawn pitbull puppies."[3] The abundant supply of puppies probably explains why as many as 18% of owners in our perception study needed to dispose of unwanted animals. With 29% of unwanted dogs being given away,[4] there is potentially a large number of recruits available to the roaming dog population. In addition to a range of "breed" puppies, potcakes are constantly available from friends, etc. As noted above, the percentage of dogs neutered in New Providence is low compared to elsewhere, and this, combined with many dogs being kept outside, makes it easy for dogs to roam and mate unchecked. Neutering is considered a key element in any programme designed to reduce or curb pet overpopulation. Increased neuter rates are said to be responsible for the decrease in the number of dogs killed by euthanasia in North America.[5]

These observations make it important to appreciate people's attitudes and actions towards neutering, or, to use the colloquial term, "fixing." An understanding of owner attitudes towards this issue is vital to inform those associated with pet education matters as well as informing neuter initiatives. Thus we feel the need to consider this issue in some detail.

A neutering campaign on one Bahamian island targeted male owners. With the slogan "Real men neuter their dogs," the sponsors assumed that men were less likely than women to have their dogs neutered[6] and singled them out as the focus of their campaign. This view was based on findings elsewhere and local observation.[7] Clearly, if the assumption was wrong, many dog owners would be excluded who should be encouraged to neuter their pets. Females might even start to feel that only male owners need to neuter their pets! Gender-related differences in attitudes of people to a number of issues related to pet dogs have been observed by us[8] and are considered to be a "common phenomenon and largely independent of culture."[9]

We have already identified some possible gender-related differences in attitudes and actions towards dogs in The Bahamas. For example, slightly fewer (p=0.08) female, 79% (of 151), than male residents, 87% (of 134), claimed to like pets "in general," but almost marginally more women (61% of 152) feed animals they do not own, compared to (52% of 133) men (p=0.12.[10] (Further differences were noted in our attachment study; see Chapter 6.)

Within Bahamian society, as elsewhere, there are gender differences concerning male intellectual superiority towards females,[11] and there are also "double standards"[12] towards acceptable sexual behaviour of males and females.[13] Bahamian men are said to fear castration, and "frequent touching of his sex organs represents . . . castration fear,"[14] so these human concerns may have contributed to a perception that men are less likely to neuter their pets. It should be noted that there may be other reasons which contribute to this fear, and elsewhere—for example, Greece—owners are reluctant to neuter their pets as a consequence of the nation's history.[15]

The study[16]

To investigate these issues we carried out a survey in 2001. A survey form was designed based upon one used in a similar study in Australia[17]; the only important differences between the forms was that ours grouped respondents by age group and asked about the ability of dogs to roam. Almost all the participants were dog owners visiting two veterinary clinics or using The College of The Bahamas library or owners contacted via a telephone study.

We use the concept of "odds ratio"[18] to identify groups which are more (or less) likely to neuter their pets. When dogs are classified in some way, for example by gender of owner, we may wish to know if there a greater percentage (i.e., "risk") of them being neutered if the dogs belong to one group (gender of owner, say) than the other. If the odds ratio is less than one, then the "risk" is less for the "first" group compared to the "second" group; if the ratio is greater than one, the reverse is true. If the 95% confidence limits of the log odds ratio includes 1, the two percentages are considered similar, and the probability of the dogs being neutered in the two groups is considered to be statistically similar.

Demographics and dog ownership

Results from 280 respondents' forms were analyzed which related to 678 dogs. Owners were classified by age (under or over 35 years of age) and class of owner (sole male, sole female, joint ownership). Thirty-one percent of respondents were sole male owners, 29% sole female owners and 38% joint owners. The percentage of younger (35 years or less) owners to older owners (over 35 years old) was similar (46% to 54%) (p=0.123), irrespective of the class of owner. The numbers of dogs owned by each class of owner were: sole male owners, 244; sole female owners, 165; and joint owners, 284. Joint owners owned more dogs than sole owners and were more likely to have neutered dogs than sole male or female owners (Table 10.4).

Gender of owner and neutering

Joint owners had a higher percentage of their dogs neutered compared to sole owners (Table 12.1). Sole males and females had a similar percentage of their dogs neutered. The closeness to one of several of the odds ratios highlights the similarity in neutering rates of animals with sole owners (Table 12.1). The odds ratio of a male dog being neutered, if it has a male owner compared to a female owner is 1.14 (95% confidence limits: 0.60–2.18), while that for a female dog is 0.77 (95% confidence limits: 0.42–1.40). Formally, these odds ratios indicate no real differences between neuter rates, although the data give the impression that men are, if anything, more likely than women to neuter male dogs.

Table 12.1: Percentage of dogs neutered and odds ratios of dogs being neutered by sole male compared with sole female owners, New Providence.

	All owners	Joint owners	Sole male owner	Sole female owner	Odds ratio	95% CL
Owners 35 years or under						
Male dogs	24	34	19	12	1.69	0.49–5.83
Female dogs	33	57	23	15	1.72	0.54–5.52
All dogs	28	45	21	13	1.71	0.73–3.98
Owners over 35 years						
Male dogs	41	41	45	32	1.74	0.81–3.74
Female dogs	65	72	57	58	0.77	0.33–1.80
All dogs	52	57	50	46	1.18	0.68–2.05
All owners						
Male dogs	34	40	33	24	1.14	0.60–2.18
Female dogs	50	66	36	42	0.77	0.42–1.40
All dogs	42	52	34	32	1.04	0.68–1.61

The higher the odds ratio, the larger the proportion of neutered dogs owned by sole males compared with the proportion of neutered dogs owned by sole females. Data, based on Fielding, Samuels & Mather (2002), are recalculated using odds ratios. CL: Confidence limits.

Age of owner and neutering of dogs

For male dogs, the odds ratio of being neutered by younger rather than older owners was 0.44 (95% confidence limits: 0.27–0.71) and for female dogs, 0.30 (95% confidence limits: 0.19–0.49). This difference was probably because 28% (of 127) younger owners wanted their animals to breed, compared with 15% of (150) older owners (p=0.012).

Whether or not a dog is neutered is strongly associated with the age of its owner. Within each owner age group, the odds ratios of a dog being neutered were similar between men and women. However, younger male owners were less likely than older men to neuter their dogs (odds ratio=0.53; 95% confidence limits 0.31–0.91); a similar result was found for female owners (odds ratio=0.18; 95% confidence limits 0.08–0.41).

Neutering and confinement of dogs

Roaming male dogs were less likely to be neutered than confined male dogs. The percentages of roaming and confined male dogs neutered were 26% (of 144) and 38% (of 214). The odds ratio of roaming male dogs being neutered, compared with those which could not roam, was 0.56 (95% confidence limits, 0.35–0.90). No similar difference was found for roaming and confined female dogs. Fifty-two percent (of 126) of confined and 53% (of 180) of roaming female dogs were neutered.

Table 12.2: Percentage of all owners, by age and owner class, who do not intend to get their animals neutered.

	Sole male	Sole female	Joint owner	All owners
35 years or under	57	54	21	45
Over 35 years	58	37	55	50
All owners	57	45	39	47

Reasons for not neutering dogs

Forty-seven percent (of 179 replies) of all owners with intact dogs did not intend to get them neutered (Table 12.2); within this group (84 replies), sole males accounted for 47% of the total and sole female owners 30%. Breeding was the most common reason for not neutering animals (Table 12.3); of those owners giving this reason, the single largest group (36% of 59 replies) was also younger males. Of the sole owners who wanted their dogs to breed, more male (79% of 28 replies) than female owners (41% of 17 replies) had no intention of getting their dogs neutered (p=0.02). Slightly more female (20%) than male (10%) owners considered neutering their dogs unnecessary (p=0.13). More female (14%) than male (2%) owners gave cost as a reason for not neutering their dogs (p=0.01). If an animal was confined, 18% of respondents thought it unnecessary to neuter it.

Table 12.3: Reasons given by owners for not neutering their pets, with the frequency with which they were reported.

Reason	Sole male owners	Sole female owners	Joint owners	Overall (%)
Want it to breed	28	17	13	32
Too young	18	12	21	29
Is fenced in	11	6	13	17
Not necessary	6	11	6	13
No reason	5	9	8	12
Did not get around to it	8	3	11	12
Cannot afford cost	1	8	9	10
Do not agree with it	4	4	4	7
May get fat	1		4	3
Sterile			3	2
Health reasons	1	2	1	2
Too old	2		1	2
Hard to catch		1	1	1
Family members will not allow it		1		1
Kept on a lead when walked		1		1
Missed previous appointment		1		1
Never thought about it	1		1	1
Changes its personality	1			1
Just found the dog	1			1
Should have right to breed		1		1
Show dog	1			1
Still thinking about it		1		1
Too close to last litter			1	1
Total number of owners	63	56	59	

Percentages of 178 owners who had intact dogs. Owners were asked to give as many reasons as they wished.

Owner attitudes towards neutering dogs

The attitudes of owners towards neutering dogs are summarized in Table 12.4. and reasons for not neutering are given in Table 12.3. There were no differences in the responses of younger and older owners to the statements listed in Table 12.4 ($p > 0.23$), so only gender aspects are considered below.

Male owners were more likely than female owners to think that female dogs should be neutered rather than male dogs (59% of men, 42% of women); that female dogs should come in heat before being neutered (41% of men, 28% of women); and neutering female dogs changes their personality (54% of men, 34% of women) (Table 12.4).

Table 12.4: Reactions of dog owners on selected aspects of their pets, percentages within each owner class.

	Agree			Disagree			Do not know			P value, all owners	P value, sole owners
	Sole male	Sole female	Joint	Sole male	Sole female	Joint	Sole male	Sole female	Joint		
Fix females rather than males to control the dog population	59	42	44	36	43	47	5	14	9	0.073	0.033
Females should come in heat before being fixed	41	28	25	39	37	49	20	35	28	0.052	0.069
Fixing a female changes its personality	54	34	27	26	33	45	20	33	28	0.002	0.034
Fixing a male dogs removes its maleness	51	30	18	38	37	57	11	33	25	<0.001	0.001
Fixing a male dog changes its personality	58	42	25	28	26	46	14	32	29	<0.001	0.018
Fixing a dog makes it sexually frustrated	38	41	22	33	34	57	29	25	21	0.005	0.859
The thought of getting my dog fixed upsets me	26	24	11	66	68	84	8	8	5	0.053	0.975
I think of my dog in human terms	70	68	61	28	25	33	2	8	6	0.378	0.237
I think of my dog's sexual needs in the same way as my own	28	30	19	56	52	71	16	18	10	0.089	0.848

Male owners were more likely than female owners to think that neutering male dogs removes their maleness (51% of men, 30% of women) and neutering male dogs changes their personality (58% of men, 42% of women) (Table 12.4).

Owner attitudes towards sexuality of their dogs

Male and female owners had similar attitudes concerning the sexuality of their dogs. Similar percentages of them were upset by the thought of neutering their dogs (26% men, 24% women); thought of the dog's sexual needs in human terms (28% men, 30% women); and thought that neutering dogs made them sexually frustrated (38% men, 41% women). A similar percentage of men and women (70% and 68% respectively) thought of their dogs in "human terms" (Table 12.4).

Sixty-six percent (of 267) of all owners thought of their dogs in human terms, and 23% *also* thought of their dogs' sexual needs in the same way as their own.

The subgroup of male owners who thought of their dogs in human terms and also thought of their dogs' sexual needs in the same way as their own had a slightly lower percentage of their *female* dogs neutered (17% of 18 dogs) than male owners in general (36%) (p=0.18). In the subgroup of owners who thought neutering a male dog removed its maleness, men had 36% (of 44 dogs) of their female dogs neutered and the women only had 14% (of 29 dogs) (p=0.023). In the same group, male owners had 23% (of 60) of their male dogs neutered, compared with 8% (of 26 dogs) of female owners (p=0.046).

Effects of attitudes on actions

The attitudes of owners towards neutering and projection of human sexuality onto their dogs were associated with differences in the percentage of dogs neutered. Table 12.5 shows that dogs are less likely to be neutered when the owner responded positively to the attitude questions, except that of considering dogs in human terms. The attitudes and associated actions were similar for both the male and female owners.

Table 12.5: Neutering percentages and odds ratios of dogs being neutered by owners in relation to attitudes about an animal's sexuality.

	Yes	No	Odds ratio	95% CL
Fixing a female changes its personality[§]	35	75	0.20	0.13–0.31
Fixing a male changes its personality[*]	28	48	0.26	0.17–0.39
Fixing a male dog removes its maleness[*]	20	48	0.33	0.22–0.50
Fixing a dog makes it sexually frustrated	32	55	0.39	0.27–0.56
The thought of getting my dog fixed upsets me	12	52	0.13	0.07–0.23
I equate a dog's sexual needs to human needs	26	47	0.41	0.27–0.64
I think of dogs in human terms	44	37	1.38	0.95–1.98

Data, based on Fielding, Samuels & Mather (2002), is recalculated using odds ratios.[*] = answers from owners of male dogs; [§] = answers from owners of female dogs.

Discussion

Interpretation of the data from any convenience sample must be made with caution, as we cannot rule out bias in the results. There was variability in some responses that depended upon where the owner's form was completed; for example, owners visiting the private veterinary clinic had 77% of their dogs neutered, compared with 38% of the dogs owned by people contacted by telephone. However, as this investigation comprised the largest ever sample of dog owners in The Bahamas, and several of its findings are in line with those found in our previous studies on dog ownership, it is hoped that any bias might not invalidate the results. For example, this study confirms that the mean number of dogs per owner is about 2.6, which we found before (p>0.18). The percentage of owners with at least one dog neutered was 45%, which is just a little higher (p=0.042) than the 40% found in our perception study in New Providence. Allowing for the fact that 23% of owners never visit the veterinarian, the adjusted number of owners who have at least one dog neutered may be closer to 35%, which matches the figure we found earlier.

Neutering aspects

Overall, 42% of all dogs in this investigation were neutered compared with 64% in Abaco, 66% in America and 77% in Australia.[19] The higher figure in Abaco probably illustrates the effect a free neuter programme can have.[20] Both in this study and Australia,[21] about 10% of owners found the cost of neutering their dogs high. In America, studies have reported 8% and 5%[22] of owners giving cost as a reason for not neutering their dogs. Our studies have shown that the cost of the neuter operation prevents people from neutering their dogs in The Bahamas (see Chapter 13), but once this barrier is removed, owners are willing to have their animals neutered, an action consistent with the attitudes shown in Table 12.4. In this study, the smaller number of owners stating cost as a reason for not getting their dogs neutered may result from a reluctance to admit their financial limitations.

The percentages of dogs neutered we reported in Chapter 10 (51% for males and 72% for females) referred to licensed animals, which form a minority of the dog population, so the lower figures in this study are probably more representative of the general dog population. (Owners who bother to license their pets might be more conscientious owners.) In Massachusetts the percentage of neutered male and female dogs was 45% and 88% respectively and in Brisbane 57% and 92% respectively.[23] These figures highlight the lower neutering rates in New Providence, 33% for males and 50% for females, particularly for female dogs.

Some side effects of neutering (increase in hunger, and decrease in activity[24]) were not specifically stated, but they might have been included when owners considered changes to a dog's "personality." Our conversations with owners show they have heard that neutered dogs are "lazy." Owners who thought that neutering might change a dog's personality appear to consider the change negatively, as they were less likely to neuter their pets (Table 12.5).

Attitudes towards neutering and sexuality

In general, owner's attitudes towards sexuality are associated with the percentage of dogs neutered (Table 12.5). Bahamian owners appear to project human values more strongly on to their dogs than other owners.[25] This attitude is also present in the press, which uses terms such as "gang rape" to describe the natural activities of dogs.[26] Viewing their dogs in human terms, combined with a willingness to consider their dogs' sexuality in a similar light as their own, probably contributes to the reluctance of Bahamians to get their dogs neutered.

However, while men felt that neutering changes a male dog's personality and removes its maleness, and they are reluctant to neuter their dogs, this did not cause them to feel upset about having their animals neutered. Despite a personal fear of castration, Bahamian men are just as likely to neuter their male dogs as sole women owners. When women report that they consider neutering a male dog removes its maleness and they fail to neuter their dogs, this may reflect gender differences in the concept of "maleness." Men may project their maleness onto their dogs but not their sexuality. Women may view their dogs as protectors (or aggressors towards enemies), a role that they feel cannot be fulfilled if the dogs' maleness or "strength" is removed through neutering. Although similar percentages of men and women (59% and 55% respectively) keep dogs for protection,[27] this might not reflect the relative importance of protection to different owners. The gender difference in attitudes indicates that in order to improve the neutering rates of pets neuter education must be gender-specific. However, the low neutering rate means that both male and female owners must be targeted in neuter campaigns.

While all three classes of owners neutered a similar proportion of male dogs, male owners had the smallest proportion of neutered female dogs. This difference is due to the fact that men breed dogs, probably for commercial purposes. No such difference was observed in Australia,[28] where commercial dog breeders form associations and follow specified codes of ethics. In The Bahamas, dog breeding is not regulated.

Many owners are ignorant about neutering. For example, a woman who had become responsible for her brother's male dog did not know whether the dog was neutered and she did not understand the terms "fixed," "sterilization," and "spay/neuter." One woman expressed the perception that male dogs "did not breed," and so there was no need to neuter them. This attitude may explain why the neuter rate of male dogs is lower for those people who allow their dogs to roam than for those that are confined.

Gender differences might not be the sole influence on actions with regard to neutering dogs. Another interpretation suggested from Table 12.3 is that there might be religious objections to neutering. In a predominantly Protestant community, such as The Bahamas, a low pet neuter rate can be expected.[29]

Reasons for not neutering

Wanting the animal to breed (32%) was the most common reason for people not having it neutered. This compares with 21% in America and 27% in Australia.[30] Ownership of dogs for breeding purposes may be more widespread in The Bahamas than elsewhere and may be related to the absence of regulations regarding dog breeding. As noted before, in the case of licensed dogs, "breed" animals are less likely to be neutered than potcakes, probably due to the value of pure-bred puppies. However, in a more general dog population, a similar proportion of dogs (p=0.18) (34% of potcakes vs. 45% of purebreds or "mixed" dogs) were neutered, irrespective of type.[31] If we assume that licensed dogs belong to more conscientious owners, it would be logical for potcake owners to neuter their dogs, as potcake puppies would be of little economic value.

In America,[32] 13% of owners cited the young age of their dog as the reason for not having it neutered, while in Australia only 5% gave this reason, compared with 29% in this study. In New Providence, the earliest age that veterinary clinics recommend that dogs should be neutered is six months, or just before first heat for females. Any delay in neutering pets is important because many dogs roam and so can produce unplanned litters; for example: one respondent complained that roaming potcakes had bred with her Chihuahua. There is a tendency in Bahamian society towards tardiness, so if owners are told to neuter their dogs at six months, they may start to make arrangements for the operation too late, which again could allow the pet to breed. For example, the person who "missed the last appointment" suggests a lack of timeliness (Table 12.3). If owners were told to neuter at four months of age, as recommended by veterinarians in other countries,[33] this might ensure that more animals were neutered before their first heat. Acceptance of the "myth" that female dogs should come in heat before being neutered (also common in North America[34]) may further encourage owners to delay the operation.

People who did not get their dogs neutered because they kept them fenced in, or on a lead (Table 12.3) may not appreciate the importance of neutering. Alternatively, owners who keep dogs in yards may consider their animals protected from roaming dogs that might otherwise harm or mate with them, and so consider neutering unnecessary. However, fences are often not stock-proof, even if they keep owned animals in. One owner who kept her dog in "a fenced yard" complained that the "strays got in, somehow, under the fence," which resulted in her dog getting pregnant.

These attitudes towards neutering are very important. If, like other attitudes towards dogs, they are entrenched and not associated with any one group of people (as is the case for some other attitudes towards dogs; see Table 13.1), then it may explain why relatively few richer dog owners have their animals neutered. We can show that all things being equal, if 80% of people who can afford to neuter their animals did so, we could expect a decrease in the number of abandoned dogs (Figure 12.1). (In this study 77% of the dogs visiting the private veterinary clinic were neutered, hence the target of 80% of dogs owned by more affluent people.) We know from personal observation that "richer" people do not necessarily maintain their fences, do not always neuter their potcakes or pure-bred dogs and can ignore the presence of flea-ridden pups in their yards.[35] The importance of these observations, combined with our estimates shown in Figure 12.1, is that it shows that "poorer" people alone are not responsible for the overpopulation problem.[36] Given the higher incomes of better-off owners, it is reasonable to have a higher expectation of them to neuter their dogs than other owners. Thus, it is clear that better-off owners alone have the potential to trigger a useful reduction in the free-roaming dog population by neutering their dogs. (Other economic issues of dog ownership are discussed in Chapter 13.)

Age aspects

Younger owners (under 35 years of age) were less inclined to have their dogs neutered than older owners (Table 12.2) due to a wish to breed them. The study also showed that the attitudes in Table 12.4 persisted irrespective of the owners' age, which suggests that previous educational efforts have failed to increase the knowledge of pet owners on the benefits of pet neutering. In recent years, animal welfare groups, veterinarians and even a yearly fun dog show[37] have probably provided more opportunities for children to learn about pet care than ever before, but participation in such events is still elective and so owners who may benefit most from these education opportunities may be absent. Peer education is still a major source of information for younger dog owners. One elderly respondent admitted that she did "not really know much about dogs." Therefore, it seems reasonable to expect that current attitudes will persist to the next generation of owners unless educational efforts are increased.[38]

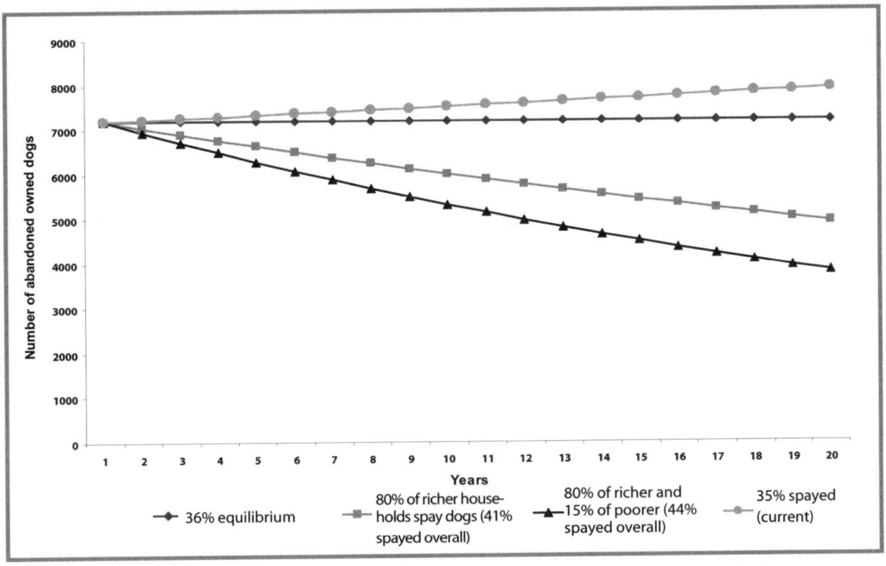

Figure 12.1: The estimated impact of various neuter rates of unowned dogs on the number of abandoned dogs.
("Richer" owners are defined to have a household income over $20,000 per year, "poorer" households have less than this amount.)

Neutering and confinement

In order to prevent unwanted litters, neutering assumes increased importance in a community that does not confine its dogs. The 42% of dogs that can roam should be considered as a minimum figure. The tendency for respondents to say that their dogs did not roam, when in fact they do, was illustrated by one of a dog's joint owners saying that the dog could not roam, while the other said that it could. In this study, the 42% of owners claiming that their dogs roam is above the 28% reported in our perception study and is, we feel, a more reliable estimate, as well as more in keeping with that which we found in Abaco.[39]

General

Figure 12.1 shows that because of the linkage between the owned and roaming populations via abandonment (shown in Table 10.16), neutering of owned dogs is an important issue, as increased levels of neutering can be expected to help reduce the number of free-roaming dogs in the long term.

There is considerable ignorance among dog owners in New Providence about neutering dogs. The fact that younger owners displayed few differences in attitudes compared with older owners suggests that education has so far failed to influence the population on pet care, and points to the importance of increased and sustained educational efforts. Since owner attitudes towards neutering and human sexuality are associated with different neuter rates of dogs, educational efforts should be focused at altering these attitudes in all groups.

The low neuter rate observed in this study appears to result from owners' identifying strongly with their pets and projecting human considerations onto them. Further work is required on how owners view sexuality so that education programmes on pet neutering can be devised to account for this and other social factors.

The fact that there is only a $4 incentive in the dog license fee to own spayed females and no incentive to neuter male dogs does not encourage owners to neuter their pets. As shown in Chapter 2, the license fees, and consequently the incentives, have fallen behind in real value and so making the cost of spaying a female unrecoverable, even if she lives to be 12 years old. Clearly, the license fee structure provides no encouragement for male dogs to be neutered. A change in the dog license fee structure might be used to provide financial gains to owners who neutered their pets, of either sex. However, such incentives will only help reduce the dog population when combined with enforcement of the Dog Licence Act.

Attitudes and actions towards neutering are not necessarily linked. No evidence could be found to support the idea than male owners were less likely than female owners to neuter their dogs. One important division between male and female owners is that young men keep dogs for breeding, and hence are unwilling to have these animals neutered. This observation suggests that the legal and ethical framework concerning dog breeding needs to be addressed in The Bahamas. Until this is done, the abundant supply of unwanted dogs (which are subsequently abandoned) can be expected to be maintained.

13

Economic Aspects of Dog Ownership

We can report that many, many well-to-do and educated folk (magistrates, church ministers and cabinet
ministers alike!!) have unspayed unkempt dogs running
the streets producing hundreds of unwanted pups![1]

Owning a dog is not without cost[2] to the owner, if the care of the animal is to exceed
that of merely giving it water and table scraps. The ability of a household to spend
money on its dogs will reflect the availability of funds and the willingness of the owners
to undertake the expense. Both aspects are important, as we know of well-to-do profes-
sional people whose level of care offered to their animals (particularly potcakes) gives
cause for concern, even though funds are not short, and we also know other owners
who, with more limited resources, offer more care.

For our purposes, we divide the population into two economic groups: "poorer"
households, which have an annual income of $20,000 or less a year; and "richer"
households, with an annual income in excess of this figure. (From the 2000 census the
median total household income was $30,200.[3])

We then classified the dog owners, in our perception study, as being "poorer" or
"richer" and we looked at a number of characteristics about their dog ownership.

Household income was not a barrier to dog ownership. Both classes of household
had a similar proportion of owning households (p=0.78), but the poorer households
(50% of our sample) owned more dogs (58% of the total) than did richer households
(p=0.03). Twenty-one percent (of 68 replies) of those in poorer households took their
pets to the clinic each year, compared with 51% (of 69 replies) of richer households
(p=0.01). Richer households were more likely to have their dogs spayed or neutered
than poorer households—58% for richer (of 60 replies) compared with 10% (of 60 replies) for poorer (p<0.001). Slightly fewer, 74% (of 62 replies), poorer people kept their
dogs in fenced-in yards, compared with 86% (of 57 replies) of richer owners (p=0.09),

and poorer households were more likely to have dogs "stolen" (p<0.001). Nuisances caused by free-roaming dogs similarly affected both richer and poorer households (p=0.81). The fact that poorer households were more likely (70% of 126 replies) to feed free-roaming dogs than richer households (46% of 125 replies) (p<0.01) may be due to the presence of community-owned dogs or the lack of stock-proof fences (Table 13.1). The pattern of responses between the poorer and richer households can be seen to reflect the comments and actions of Miss F and Mr. M. in the case studies in Chapter 7. The similarity in responses from households with different economic status may suggest that many attitudes are deeply rooted (cultural?) and not necessarily socio-economically related. These observations indicate that educational efforts at enhancing dog welfare must be aimed at all sections of society.

One question which these statistics raise is why so many richer households have intact dogs. If these animals are kept for breeding, what happens to the puppies? The impact of intact dogs from richer households on the abandoned population has already been illustrated (Figure 12.1). Possibly, there is a high mortality rate in the litters and the survivors are used to replace dead adults or given away.

Although about 75% of richer owners claim that their dogs do not roam, 25% admit they do allow them to roam. This means that richer owners could be allowing some 9,000 dogs to roam. Given that the number of people who admit to their dogs roaming is probably less than the number who do, richer people could be responsible for an even greater number of dogs roaming and so also contribute even more to the maintenance of the free-roaming dog population. This again shows that the roaming dog problem should not be simply thought of as a poor person's problem.

Table 13.1: Indicators of animal welfare by household income of owner, New Providence.

	% Poorer households n~68	% Richer households n~69
Like pets in general	85	83
Keep dogs in a "fenced" yard	74	86
Have dogs stolen	31	7
Have dogs which roam	30	25
Take their pet to the vet yearly	21	51
Have licensed dogs	20	31
Dispose of unwanted dogs	16	21
Have neutered dogs	10	58
Would dispose of unwanted animals inhumanely	10	6

Note: the sample size, n, was not the same for each question. Poorer households have incomes under $20,000 per year, richer households exceed this amount.

The pattern of disposal of unwanted animals by economic class of household is given in Table 13.2, but the sample size is too small to allow us to show any significant differences between poorer and richer households. However, superficial examination suggests that poorer households may be more likely to abandon animals,[4] while richer households are more likely to have pets killed by euthanasia. The occurrence of "stolen" animals may be higher in poorer households (Table 13.2), as they are less able to contain their pets. However, from our own observations, many yards, in both economic groups, which owners claim are stock-proof do not actually stop dogs from getting in or out. Gates are often left open, particularly for the convenience of getting in and out by car, and where more than one household shares a yard, keeping fence gates closed is even more difficult. Thus, it is possible that dogs which merely wander off and do not return or get killed by cars might be considered stolen. While such animals might be reported as stolen, they may be recruits to the unowned roaming dog population. If this is so, the number of recruits may be higher than we have reported above.

Table 13.2: Summary of methods used to dispose of unwanted animals by households classified by household income.

Method of disposal	% Poorer households (n=17)	% Richer households (n=22)
Abandon	41	18
To humane group	24	36
Euthanasia	12	23
Give away	12	9
Animal Control Unit	12	9
Shoot	0	5

Poorer households have incomes under $20,000 per year, richer households exceed this amount.

While all groups need to be encouraged to confine and neuter their pets, it might be argued that given their economic situation it would be reasonable that the educational emphasis for poorer households should be to encourage the surrender of unwanted animals. "Giving away" dogs, while convenient, and possibly considered more "humane" to the owner than surrendering, is no guarantee that the animal is disposed of in a humane way and/or prevents it from joining the free-roaming population.

Dog owning households own about 2.5 dogs each, which is more than the number owned in some other countries, and this places a greater burden on Bahamian households if they wish to provide adequate pet care. The presence of so many dogs in the household can be explained by the ease with which dogs can be acquired (potcake puppies are available year-round and are typically given away[5]), and the fact that many people want several dogs to run in the yard in order to protect their property. (Owners are almost encouraged, or it is at least expected, to have two dogs in their yard, and leaders of society see nothing wrong in this behaviour; see Chapter 16.)

We have little information concerning the amount of money that owners spend on keeping a dog. Preliminary information from the Bahamas Humane Society suggests that, in 1993, households with dogs spent an average of about $52 on clinic fees. If the dogs are fed manufactured dog food, this would cost in the region of $550 per animal/year, and essential medicines, such as heartworm tablets, etc., would cost an additional $109 per animal/year, so the cost per household could be in the region of $1,800/year. This would represent a large sum for a household earning less than $20,000 per year. Thus, it is understandable that poorer households might not be able to spend as much on health care as richer households.

If inadequate dog ownership is considered as a "crime," then it can be argued that changes in the behaviour of richer owners would not only be beneficial to society in the short term, but would also encourage changes in the way poorer people own dogs in the long term.[6] One clear "crime" concerns non-compliance with the dog licensing law. The majority of both richer and poorer owners do not license their pets. If richer owners licensed their dogs, this would be an important step to providing peer pressure on poorer owners to accept the duties associated with pet ownership. Richer owners could use their influence to encourage enforcement of the law but this cannot be achieved when their behaviour is not much different from the poorer owners'. Regretfully, as we saw earlier, richer households have historically been reluctant to comply with dog-related taxes. Likewise, richer owners could take the lead in confining their dogs. It has already been shown (in Figure 12.1) that if more of the richer owners neutered their animals, a reduction in the roaming dog population could be expected. Although a greater decrease could be expected if more of the poorer owners neutered their animals, the peer pressure on poorer owners is lacking, due to the inaction of richer owners. Thus, the role of richer owners might be crucial in bringing about changes in animal welfare in less affluent households.

Packs of dogs on beaches give tourists a negative impression of New Providence.

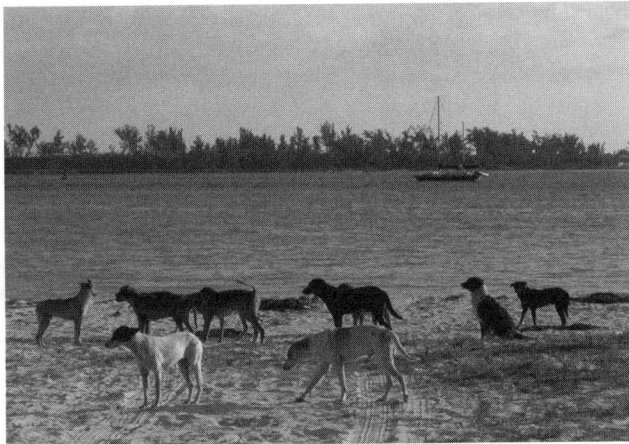

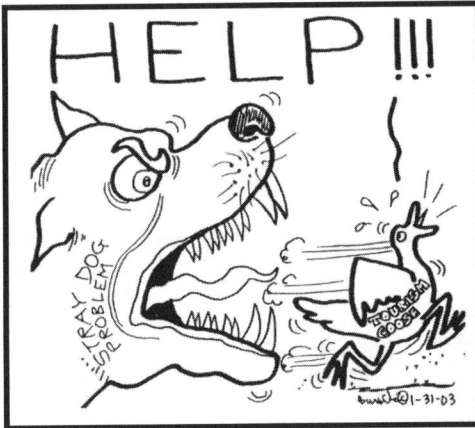

This cartoon in *The Tribune* newspaper indicates the national concern that roaming dogs can be a threat to the most important industry in The Bahamas. (Courtesy of Stanley Burnside)

Sick dogs cause offense and so are remembered, even if they are not very common. Such a dog could have been the genesis of Fleabag.

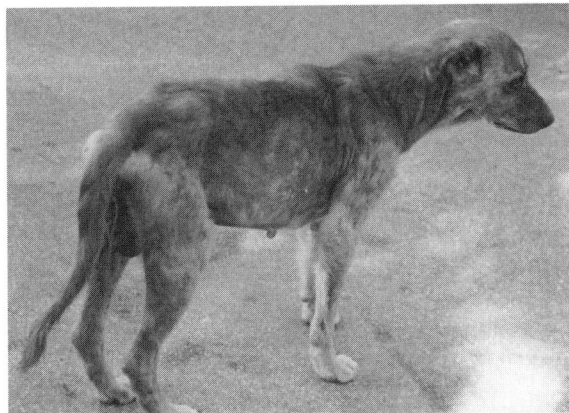

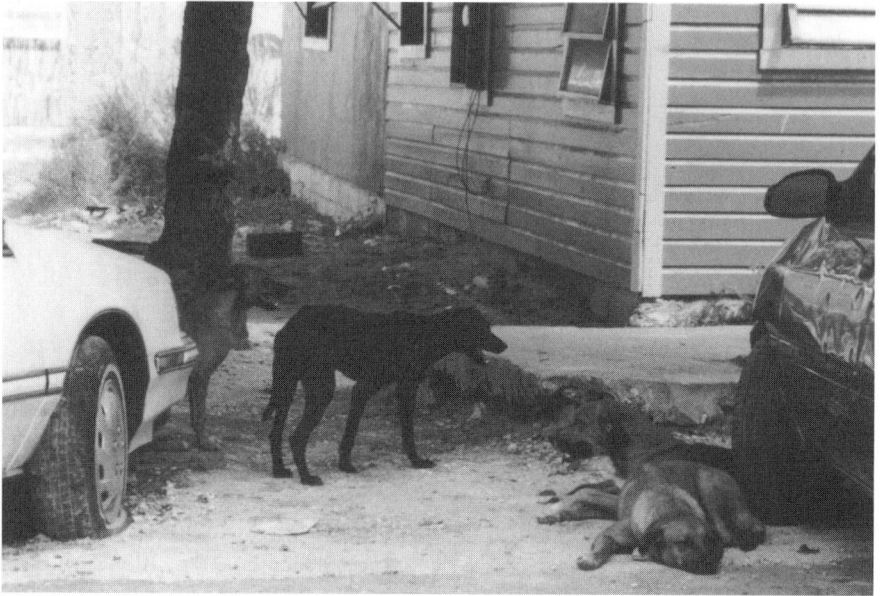

Roaming dogs are most common in poorer neighbourhoods, where they may be community-owned due to a lack of fenced-in yards.

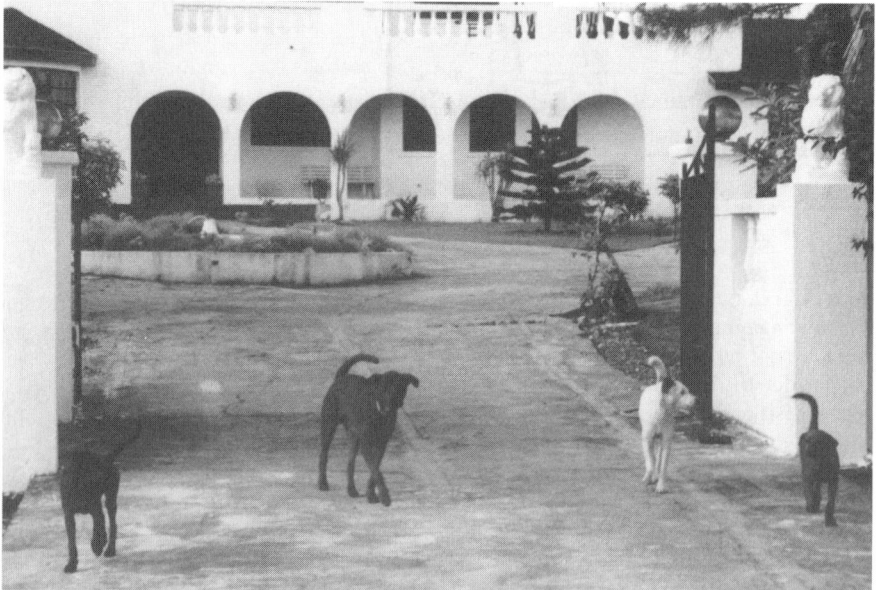

Many roaming potcakes are owned. Even in high-class districts owners allow their dogs to roam, possibly because they think the dogs can better protect the home.

14

Cruelty to Dogs

He [His Excellency in 1924] did not believe that there were many cases of intentional cruelty."[1]

We [Bahamas Humane Society Officers] have seen really sadistic treatment of animals.[2]

These two quotations from the press, despite their contradictory messages, are probably both true. Since 1841, society has required that animals be treated kindly, and this long-standing demand has been reflected in the presence of groups championing the "rights"[3] of animals from the 1890s and the current law. The Penal Code, quoted below, prohibits the abuse of animals and deals with cruelty to animals by laying down basic conditions under which animals must be kept. Shade, food and water are also required for animals, and animals cannot be used or transported so that they are harmed:

> Whoever intentionally and unlawfully kills, maims or wounds an animal . . . which is of some value, and which is and appears tamed, is domesticated or is in a state of actual confinement, shall be liable to imprisonment . . .

and

> Whoever cruelly beats, ill-treats, starves, overrides, overdrives, overloads, abuses, tortures or otherwise maltreats an animal of any species . . . shall be guilty of an offence . . .[4]

The law also requires animals to be kept in a "clean, comfortable and sanitary condition."[5] As indicated earlier, The Bahamas has long been concerned that animals (particularly horses) are well treated, and many organizations and people have been involved in putting their concern into practice.

Of the four types of "cruelty" ("cruel," "abuse," "neglect" and "use"[6]) we consider "cruelty" in the context of intentional acts (abuse); unintentional harm is usually the result of animal neglect and owner ignorance (neglect). Elsewhere it has been found that judgments of cruelty towards animals are not simple, and appear to depend upon

the gender of the judger, the gender of the person causing the cruelty and the circumstances under which the act is performed.[7] Apart from one student study,[8] there seems
to be little systematically collected information on animal abuse in New Providence, so
it is necessary to rely upon information from welfare groups, newspaper reports and
our own experience.

Apart from the occasional use of dogs for illegal gain and maltreatment of training
"bad dogs," criminals sometimes kill or harm dogs.[9] The use of dogs for household security might cause dogs to be hurt in one-third of attacks on homes with dogs.[10] Owned
dogs which residents consider a nuisance can also be abused.[11] In the case of unowned
dogs, we feel that the most common act of intentional harm is poisoning, while in the
case of owned dogs neglect, poisoning and abandonment are probably the most common. In fact, the press, presumably unintentionally, has actually described how to poison
dogs![12] Acts of harm typically rise after adverse publicity associated with dogs,[13] which is
an understandable response when people fear for their personal safety. Regrettably, allega-
tions concerning the poisoning of owned potcakes have been reported in the foreign
press.[14] Owners' ever-increasing consciousness of their pets' welfare is illustrated by concerns about the possible harm that the irresponsible use of fireworks may cause their
dogs.[15] However, the Bahamas Kennel Club feels that in the last 40 years "there has not
been much improvement" in the area of animal "cruelty."[16]

Veterinarians, as well as Bahamas Humane Society officers, watch for and report
cases of intentional harm. In the first five months of 2000, about five cases of animal
"cruelty" were brought before the courts[17]; however, it should be noted that the Bahamas is not alone in rarely punishing abusers.[18]

Although the majority of residents like pets and feel sorry for free-roaming
dogs, some are still harmed, and the Bahamas Humane Society estimates that 95%
of "cruelty reports" concern potcakes.[19] Consequently, potcakes would appear to
bear the brunt of cruelty towards dogs.

"Cruelty" towards roaming dogs

We believe a major reason for this rises from frustration when residents are unable to
get nuisance dogs removed. Although there is a long-established humane society in
Nassau, it is not responsible for collection of stray animals[20] and the government's
Animal Control Unit is limited in its capacity and so cannot always provide the trapping service which some would like.[21] (The Unit does not normally catch dogs between
4.00 p.m.–8.00 a.m. or on weekends and holidays, so catching opportunities are limited.) It should also be noted that the Unit is sometimes prevented from collecting dogs
by residents,[22] thus adding to the frustration of those who wish to have the dogs removed. Understandably, reports in the press have focused on the use of poison to kill
dogs, or acid to inflict pain.[23] Even dog owners can get fed up with roaming dogs and
resort to inhumane removal of these animals; "I had to take care of them myself," admitted one dog owner who had poisoned roaming dogs. Some nuisance dogs have

been shot by people wanting to sleep at night.[24] However, interviews with residents suggest that few people take more aggressive action than either "shooing" the dog from the yard or throwing a stone.

However, actions taken against dogs often indicate unwillingness by residents to confront owners of roaming or nuisance animals. This unwillingness often arises from the close-knit and stable nature of many communities. Neighbours may be unable or unwilling (often due to family or business ties) to approach owners about the dog's behaviour, so they may take action against the dog. Possibly for similar reasons there is also reluctance by residents to be witnesses in cruelty cases, which prevents prosecution of alleged perpetrators.[25]

However, given the size of the dog populations, and that many people are not dog owners, the frequency of harm to dogs is probably low, although 46% of the respondents in our perception study considered roaming dogs as a nuisance. In Bain Town and Yamacaw, 57% and 83% (each of 35 respondents)[26] claimed to have suffered "violent attacks" by roaming dogs, so making roaming dogs a personal threat in these areas. This worry could understandably result in residents' protecting themselves as best they can.

A student's study on "cruelty" towards dogs collected views from 117 students (23% male) with a mean age of 20.7 years (se=0.51). Ninety-four percent of these respondents had roaming dogs in their neighbourhood and they had seen a mean of 5.5 (se=0.48) roaming dogs the day before. While 29% thought that the animals were "unacceptably" treated by residents, 21% thought the animals were "acceptably" treated, with the remainder being "unsure." Eighty-one percent of respondents (of 46 replies) who said their neighbours' or community dogs roamed considered such behaviour unacceptable. So although many people allow their dogs to roam, this is considered unacceptable to all except 11% of their neighbours, who thought it acceptable; the remainder were unsure.[27]

The most common reasons given for dogs' being "unacceptably" treated indicated that the dogs were targets of abuse from people throwing rocks[28] at them or poisoning them. Fifty percent of respondents considered feeding unowned dogs acceptable and 38% unacceptable (the remainder were unsure of their feeling). (This is broadly consistent with the 53% of respondents in our perception study who fed dogs they did not own.) When dogs bark at night, 51% of respondents did "nothing" and 13% did something other than speak to the owner. When dogs tip over garbage, the most common action would be to improve the storage of the garbage (49%), while 9% would do nothing, 22% would speak to the owner and the remainder would do something else. However, despite this tolerance to the nuisances of roaming dogs, 80% had heard about people harming dogs and 77% had, at some time, witnessed actions of "harm" towards dogs, the single most common act being hitting or beating dogs (35% of 91 responses), but 56% of respondents had seen acts of poisoning, starvation, neglect and/or physical violence. Although some respondents felt poisoning and/or killing to be cruel, 3% admitted that they would still poison or kill dogs which were a nuisance.

"Cruelty" towards owned dogs

In the case of owned dogs, the Bahamas Humane Society officers say neglect is the major cause of harm to the animals.[29] In a student's study on "cruelty"[30] 88% of the owned dogs were potcakes. That study found that 90% (of 40 owners) kept their dogs outside and 43% allowed them to roam, while only 13% provided them with shelter.

The actions that respondents in the cruelty study considered to constitute "cruelty" are listed in Table 14.1. These replies illustrate a wide range of actions, from those which are clearly inhumane and illegal (abuse, poisoning) to those which show some respondents to be very sensitive as to what constitutes "cruelty." The fact that while neglect was widely considered cruel yet at the same time is the most common form of cruelty may result from a lack of awareness or education as to what is adequate pet care. Interestingly, these responses inadvertently show the wide level of care which Bahamian owners do offer their animals. Pets that get baths and grooming are clearly enjoying a lifestyle different from those confined outside on a short chain.

Table 14.1: Actions considered as "cruelty" towards dogs.

Action	% of respondents
General neglect, e.g. starvation, lack of health care	70
Hitting with rocks/beating, etc.	51
Abuse (unspecified)	19
Poisoning	17
Hit by car on purpose	9
Abandonment	7
Burning*/Acid	6
Not showing dog affection	5
Allowing dogs to roam	4
Confining to small area	3
Fighting dogs	3
Killing (unspecified)	3
Drowning	2
Keeping dogs on a short tether	2
Shooting	1
Feeding peppery food	1
Using pepper spray	1
Not grooming dogs	1
Not helping dogs after being hit by a car	1
Leaving dogs defenseless	1
Not bathing dogs	1
Not taking dogs for walks	1

One-hundred and seven respondents suggested actions which they considered cruel. Respondents were allowed to nominate as many actions as they wished.[31]
*This may mean by fire or acid.

About 31% of owners in our perception study had needed to dispose of unwanted animals. Of these, 11% had done so inhumanely; such methods included
abandoning and shooting (but we also know that animals are drowned). In the cruelty
study, 9.4% (of 115 respondents) either would abandon or had abandoned animals
they did not want, while 37% would give the animals away if they could. If respondents
saw a dog with a painful wound, 37% (of 116 replies) would leave the dog, and 9.6%
would help the dog themselves, while 51% would call the Bahamas Humane Society.

The final act of neglect towards an animal is abandonment. As indicated in Table
10.16, abandonment is the main source of animals to the roaming dog population.
While abandonment is most common for potcakes, pure-bred dogs are also abandoned. We feel that many people prefer to abandon a dog in order to "give it chance"
rather than surrender the animal, but we have not yet determined just how common
this attitude might be. This attitude is exemplified by a couple who found puppies belonging to their neighbour in their yard. The neighbour denied responsibility for the
puppies, so the couple then debated between themselves about where they should leave
the puppies; it seems to have been agreed or understood that they would not surrender
the dogs to an animal welfare group. Such attitudes can superficially appear to be kind
(life is better than death; "give it a chance"), but they show the need for educating non-
owners to appreciate the kind of life to which they are consigning abandoned dogs.

The study on "cruelty"[32] found that 60% of all respondents were aware that people promoted dogfights, and 77% (of 73 replies) found this unacceptable, 14% acceptable and the remainder was unsure. This suggests that despite the activity being illegal,
there is a core of dog owners (11% of 27 replies) who find it acceptable and may participate in it, as they found it "good entertainment." Also a 21-year-old male respondent wrote on his questionnaire: "Dog fighting is acceptable to me if both dogs are
trained to fight or have been breed for fighting, but if a defenseless dog that wasn't
trained to fight has to defend itself against a dog that is, then its unacceptable, or even if
both dogs weren't breed for fighting then its unacceptable."

One reason why owners continue to keep dogs in ways that may give cause for
concern is linked with the unwillingness of residents to confront neighbours and exert
pressure on owners to change their level of care.[33] Owners who have may have "lost"
dogs or had them poisoned by neighbors frustrated by the actions of the dogs can easily
acquire more animals and continue to keep the new ones in the same way.

Thirty-seven percent of respondents in Bain Town and 46% in Yamacraw thought
that owners allowed dogs to roam because it was cruel to confine them.[34] This attitude
and associated behaviour might also be linked to the observation that "no one ever
seems to notice the children who are often wandering about too—both in and out of
school hours,"[35] which suggests that dog owners might also fail to monitor their children. This issue requires further investigation in a society with many roaming dogs that
might be at risk to acts of harm, as indeed would be the case for unsupervised children.

There are well-established links between "cruelty" to animals and humans.[36] No studies on this issue have been done in The Bahamas, but Bahamas Humane Society officers know of at least two males who harmed dogs; one man was then killed in an armed robbery and the other arrested for causing grievous bodily harm to a relation, so such linkages also appear to be present in Bahamian society:

> Over the years I [a Bahamas Humane Society officer] have identified students who are going to be a nuisance to society just by their treatment of animals. When I check their background, they are generally from abusive families.[37]

> Children and animals are much the same, dependent on their parents or owners for their survival. What they become depends on how they are treated.[38]

A study of Bahamian schoolchildren indicates that at least 18%[39] of children suffered emotional or verbal abuse by adults in the household, at least 13% had suffered physical abuse from adults in the household and at least 2.5% had been sexually abused by adults in the household. The same study found that at least 56% of youth had thought of killing someone. These figures suggest that child abuse is present within households, and so these children may become future abusers of animals or people.[40] Reports indicating that child abuse and neglect cases are apparently increasing[41] may be warnings that animal abuse and neglect might also be increasing.

Obviously, all animal "cruelty" is to be condemned, but a few well-publicized incidences[42] should neither be interpreted as indicating that "cruelty" towards animals is widespread or part of Bahamian culture nor that Bahamians are alone in harming animals.[43] In the United Kingdom, neglect and abandonment of dogs accounted for 86% of convictions obtained by the Royal Society for the Prevention of Cruelty to Animals during 1990–1992.[44] This indicates that the problems seen in The Bahamas are similar to those seen elsewhere, even in a so-called "nation of dog lovers," Britain.[45]

The Humane Society of Grand Bahama feels that "the public is getting the message and do care about the animals,"[46] particularly as concerns abandoning dogs, which indicates that the public in general is indeed concerned about animal welfare. The examples and data given above indicate that education and law enforcement are key to reducing acts of harm towards dogs. Perceptions such as those relating to it being right or wrong to allow dogs to roam are particularly important, as they indicate some of the barriers which animal welfare educationists must face. As indicated earlier, welfare groups do participate in the education of children on animal welfare, but it is clear that peer actions undermine its effect. As long as the resources of welfare groups remain inadequate, they will be unable to sustain a systematic animal welfare programme in schools. It would appear that until a comprehensive and sustained educational programme is implemented which accounts for cultural sensitivities and targets schools in particular, dogs and especially potcakes may continue to be abused.

15

Health Issues Related to Dogs

> The harsh fact is that wild dogs are a danger to our
> health and a potential threat to the country's economy.
> Bacteria in dog faeces can cause blindness in children—
> and worms transmitted by dogs can lead to serious
> stomach and kidney ailments.[1]

As noted previously, the media have contained many reports that suggest that roaming dogs (potcakes) are a major health risk to residents. A casual reading of these statements, which can be expected when people scan newspapers, leaves the impression that dogs are a great "danger" to human health. Such reports are probably major sources of the widespread concern that we found residents had of catching diseases from dogs. However, although the human population must be at some risk of catching diseases from dogs, it is important to put these risks in perspective so that people can better assess the likelihood of the "danger" they face from dogs. Rather than making people think that they will catch diseases from dogs, dogs should be thought of as co-sufferers of these diseases.[2] To make people scared of dogs is to almost invite residents to fear and so attack the animals in order to protect their personal health.

An interesting illustration of ambivalence or ignorance on roaming dogs and health is shown at some schools. At a school attended by WF's daughter, roaming potcakes frequented the grounds[3] and quadrangles, apparently without staff interference. Allowing dogs access to school grounds unnecessarily increases the risks of a vulnerable age group of catching diseases.[4] Further, the presence of roaming dogs also provided "entertainment" for the schoolboys, who "enjoy frightening off" the animals.[5]

Health issues other than dog bites

Although there are some 65 diseases that people can catch from dogs, dogs are not necessarily the sole vector of these disorders.[6] Previously, we noted that the free-roaming

125

dog population is unhealthy. However, it was seen that the low age of owned dogs, combined with the fact that many owned dogs never visit the veterinarian, could also mean that many owned dogs are also unhealthy.[7] Humans do not ordinarily come into close contact with roaming dogs, as such dogs keep their distance and often retreat when a person approaches, as first described in 1888. Owned dogs may pose a greater health hazard to humans due to their closer proximity than roaming dogs, but with many owned dogs being kept outside the house, there may be less direct contact between dog and owner than one might first think. However, it should be noted that contact with pets can have beneficial effects for human health by reducing the incidence of allergies.[8]

In 2001, we carried out a study with the Department of Public Health to estimate the incidences of four dog-related diseases and dog bites. The diseases chosen were Scabies, *Toxocara* spp., *Leptospirosis*, and *Cutaneous larval migrans*, as they were known to be present in the dog population.[9] From our 1998 study, we know that poorer households own more dogs than richer households and are less likely to keep their dogs in a fenced-in yard, less likely to take their pets to the veterinarian and more likely to feed dogs which they do not own than richer owners. Consequently, poorer people could be expected to be at a greater risk than richer people of suffering disorders related to dogs.[10] Given this background, the population of patients we investigated was those visiting public health clinics. Clients of these clinics tend to be poorer members of society,[11] and this population was studied in order to increase the chance of detecting relevant disorders. The Ministry of Health allowed only doctors to interview patients. This meant that the completeness of interviews was dependent upon the workload of the doctors. This constraint resulted in gaps in the information required by the study; as a result the likely cause of disorders in patients was not always determined.

Six-hundred and forty-eight patients were screened during the study. Sixty-five percent (of 535 responses) of the patients were female. The overall median age was 21 years (range: 0.17–84 years) (of 367 patients). The female median age was 25 (of 213 records) and the male median age 16 years (of 153 records); thus the males were younger than the females (p<0.001). Thirty-two percent (of 97 records) of patients lived in dog-owning households and 57% (of 97 records) had stray dogs visiting their yards.[12] Thirty-six percent (of 96 records) of patients paid (at least) weekly visits to households with dogs. Seventy-five percent (of 106 replies) of patients had dogs in their yard or visited dog-owning households. Fifty-four percent (of 101 records) of patients lived in households where rodents were present. Thirty-eight percent (of 101 replies) had both rodents and dogs in their yards. Thus many patients visiting the clinics can be considered to live in close proximity to dogs. Ten patients also owned cats; of these 40% also had rodents in or around their dwellings.

The numbers of patients per 1,000 visiting the clinics because of disorders related to selected animal complaints are given in Table 15.1.

Table 15.1: Summary of the incidence of selected animal related disorders observed in two public health clinics, New Providence.

Complaint	Observed incidents per 1,000
Scabies	43
Toxocara spp.	0
Leptospirosis	0
Cutaneous larval migrans	0
Dog bites	15

648 patients were screened in the study.

No patient (12 records) with scabies owned a dog, but two patients with scabies had dogs with mange in their yard.[13] One patient with scabies owned a cat. Thus two, or 0.69:1,000 of all patients, may have caught scabies directly from dogs. Fifty-five percent (of 11 records) of patients had rodents in their yard and 28% (of 14 records) of patients had stray dogs visiting their yard. Sixty-six percent (of 11 records) of patients visited households with dogs. Fifty-nine percent of patients (of 17 records) had dogs visiting their yard or visited households with dogs. The median age of patients with scabies was eight years of age (range: 11 months–32 years), suggesting that children are most at risk. The median female and male ages were similar, at nine and six years, respectively. Seventy-five percent (of 28 records) of the patients with scabies were females, a proportion of females similar to that in the entire patient population (p>0.20).

No patient had *Toxocara spp., Leptospirosis,* or *Cutaneous larval migrans.*

Dog bites

Ten patients suffered dog bites, one of whom was certainly bitten by his own dog. The cause of the other dog bites was not reported, but one bitten patient also owned six dogs. The median age of those bitten was 18.5 years (range: 12–51) (six records); six of those bitten were females with a median age of 15 years (five records) and the only male age recorded was 44 years. The ratio of female to male victims reflects the overall use of the clinics by gender.

Discussion

As with all disorders, there is a risk of under-reporting, as not everyone seeks medical treatment/advice even though they suffer ill-health. As a result, the data may be conservative in reflecting the actual occurrences of these conditions. The study was conducted for a limited period of time, and it is not known if the time of year could have influenced the results. It should also be recalled that the population in this study was largely composed of poorer residents, who might be regarded as being at greater risk from dog-related disorders than the population as a whole.

When trying to observe rare events, the lack of a positive identification does not mean that the event is actually absent in the population. When a disorder was not observed, the maximum rate of the disorder is calculated based upon the sample size and using a 95% confidence level; as the sample size increases, the maximum incidence rate decreases.[14] Given the population of The Bahamas, when no disorder is observed, the maximum likely (95% confidence level) incidence rate is 0.01:1,000.

Scabies

The observed incidence was 28:648 or 43:1,000. Between 1990 and 1999, the average yearly incidence of scabies in all The Bahamas was 0.29:1,000, but the year-to-year incidence ranged from 0 to 1.1:1,000; hence it has a high year-to-year variability. Doctors at the study clinics were of the view that the disorder was transmitted between school children. Reports of occasional outbreaks of scabies in schools have been reported in the press.[15] The vulnerability of children to contracting scabies would account for the low median age of the patients (eight years), compared with that of the patient population (21 years), and the year-to-year variability would probably reflect localized outbreaks. Where recorded, no patient with scabies lived in a household owning dogs, so this suggests a weak link between owned dogs and scabies in humans. However, it is possible that the disorder could be introduced into schools by roaming dogs or by pupils from dog "owning" households.[16]

Toxocara spp., Leptospirosis, Cutaneous larval migrans

Although we observed no cases of these disorders in 648 patients, we cannot be certain that the incidence rate is 0:648 or less than 1.5:1,000. Given the sample size, we can be, statistically speaking, 95% confident that the rate does not exceed 4.6:1,000. In the 10-year period 1990–1999, only two cases of *Leptospirosis* were reported in all The Bahamas, so the yearly average can be estimated at 0.0019:1,000.[17] Only a blood test can give a definitive diagnosis of *Leptospirosis,* so it is not always detected in a consultation, and thus can easily be under-reported. Only an intensive study can definitively assess the prevalence of *Leptospirosis.* As neither this study nor others from The Bahamas reported any incidences of *Toxocara spp.* or *Cutaneous larval migrans,* it would suggest that the incidence rates for these disorders is less than the 4.6:1,000 we derived in this study. In 1998, the Public Health clinics in New Providence reported 73 new cases of skin and subcutan tissue problems (other than scabies), and so if we make the (probably unfair) assumption that all these were due to larval migrans, its incidence would not exceed 0.43:1,000.[18]

Dog bites

Other than the physical injury suffered from dog bites, we feel that patients probably visit the doctor because they are concerned about tetanus, not rabies. However, we feel that the absence of serious zoonotic diseases such as rabies may result in underreporting of dog bites.

We found 10:648 instances of dog bites, which gives an incidence of 15:1,000. One patient was bitten by his own dog, but the other records do not allow us to establish whether owned or unowned dogs were responsible for most of these injuries. Our perception study showed that an equal proportion of both men and women own dogs (p>0.10). A greater proportion of females (62% of 151 replies) than males (51% of 134 replies) (p=0.055) feed unowned dogs (despite women being less associated with dogs than men are). There seems to be little evidence to suppose that women are really more concerned than men about stray dogs as a health hazard, as broadly similar proportions (72% of 87 replies) of females and (61% of 134 replies) males (p=0.093) expressed this concern. In this study, although six females and four males were bitten, the sample size is too small to detect any gender bias.

Studies elsewhere have shown that over 80% of bite victims were familiar with the dog that bit them and children who own a dog are about twice as likely to be bitten as those who do not own a dog.[19] Others have reported a median age of 15 years for dog bite victims,[20] which is reasonably similar to the median age in this study, suggesting that younger people are at a higher risk. It has also been reported that 58% of dog bites occurred at home,[21] which confirms the idea that owned dogs are mainly responsible for bites. Our 1998 study indicated that a greater proportion (67% of 125 replies) of poorer residents were concerned about catching diseases from stray dogs than richer people (46% of 125 replies) (p=0.052). As our study probably focused on poorer Bahamians, who might be more at risk from being bitten than others, and with their greater concern about catching diseases from dogs, we might have found relatively minor bites being presented at public clinics. However, it would be reasonable to consider Bahamian dog owners to be at a greater risk of dog bites than those in other countries where households own fewer dogs.[22]

Despite 75% of the patients at the two public health clinics being in close proximity to dogs, less than 6% of them had contracted any disorder that could be directly associated with dogs. It is clear from Table 15.1 that although people visited the clinics with disorders that can be caught from dogs, apart from dog bites themselves, there were only two incidences which linked the disorders and dogs, and both animals were unowned. However, it should not be automatically assumed that the dogs passed on the disorders to the patients. Although scabies was the most common of the disorders investigated, dogs appear to be an uncommon vector.

It should also be noted than many patients at the public clinics had rodents (rats and/or mice) in close proximity to their households, and so rodents may pose an even greater health hazard than dogs. The fact that some people leave dog food accessible to rats may allow the rat population to increase.[23] Different species of rats and mice are associated with different *Leptospirosis* serovars (or types) and some cause more serious disease in people than others. In New Providence, the rats and mice commonly seen about houses are the Norwegian rat (*Rattus novegicus*), the roof rat (*Rattus rattus*) and the house mouse (*Mus musculus*).[24] The proximity of dogs and rodents in almost 40% of patient households might be considered a more dangerous combination to the public than either alone. The fact that some cat owners also had rodents in their yards shows that the presence of a cat is insufficient to rid households of vermin, possibly because dogs are preventing the cats from catching rodents.

A public health issue of concern is that dogs can facilitate vectors, such as mosquitoes, by scattering garbage. For example, lunch box containers can hold water after rain and become breeding sites for mosquitoes. These could then encourage outbreaks of mosquito-related diseases.

These observations seem to undermine the rationale behind the flow of public messages cautioning the population about catching diseases from dogs and in particular from "stray" or "wild" dogs. The incidence rates, although they confirm that it is possible to contract these disorders, also suggest that the warnings in the media about dogs being a public health hazard may be a tactic to manufacture headlines rather than inform the public about real dangers. Comparison of the risk figures in Table 15.1 with the risk of other disorders in The Bahamas shows that obesity is almost 10 times more common than Scabies and that traffic accidents are twice as common as dog bites.[25] Thus, there are far greater threats to people's health than dogs. Even in the context of rabies control, only one human death from rabies was reported in Florida between 1995–1999, which again shows that the risk of catching this disease can be slight. (Even in this case it is not known if a dog was responsible for the person contracting rabies.[26]) Basic human hygiene and the provision of good pet care should all but eliminate the risk of humans getting disorders from dogs.[27] The occurrence of these disorders in the human population may indicate a need for better education of human hygiene and preventive health care.

While the consequences of residents' fear about catching disorders from dogs are hard to quantify, it is possible to speculate that such fear can encourage acts of cruelty towards dogs as people try to ensure that dogs stay away from them.

The incidences of dog-related disorders require that this study be repeated on a larger scale and also to include more complaints (e.g., Campylobacter, salmonella and allergy). Further detailed investigations, in more locations, and over longer periods should be conducted to examine the direct and indirect effects of dogs on human health in The Bahamas and their interaction with wild animals associated with households.

16

Dog Bites

The Bahamian potcake has mixed with many larger and ferocious breeds of dogs such as the Doberman pinscher, German Shepherd and Pitbull, which make these packs of free-roaming dogs even more dangerous.[1]

Dog bites are the only undisputed injury which dogs can inflict on people, and we consider them further here. We also examine some of the responses of society to fatal attacks by dogs on residents.

In addition to the information on dog bites obtained in the study cited in Chapter 15, data from the public hospital in Nassau, the Princess Margaret Hospital, were obtained on dog bites reported during the period 1990 to 2001.[2] In-patient as well as out-patient data were available, so that more severe bites could be distinguished from lesser ones.

During the period 1990–2001, the mean number of patients[3] bitten by dogs per year was 192.8 (se=33.88), with a maximum of 402 and a minimum of 52. Considerable year-to-year variability is seen in the data (Figure 16.1), but the three-year moving average, which smoothes out yearly fluctuations, indicates a general upward trend (the linear regression slope is significantly non-zero at p=0.023), despite a recent decline in cases since 1998. A slight upward trend would be expected as the populations, both dog and human, increase, but smoothed data (three-year moving averages) suggest an increase of about 4% per year from 1991–2000, which is above the increase in population growth.

Admissions data (indicator of more serious dog bite injuries[4])

During the period 1989–2000, the mean number of admissions per year was six (se=1.101) with a maximum of 13 and a minimum of 2 (Figure 16.2). Although there was no linear trend in the data, the number of admittances has been rising since 1995, but the number for 2000 (12) was almost the same as that in 1990 (13). The pattern in admittances is consistent with a quadratic relationship over time (all coefficients, p<0.024) that increases post-1995.

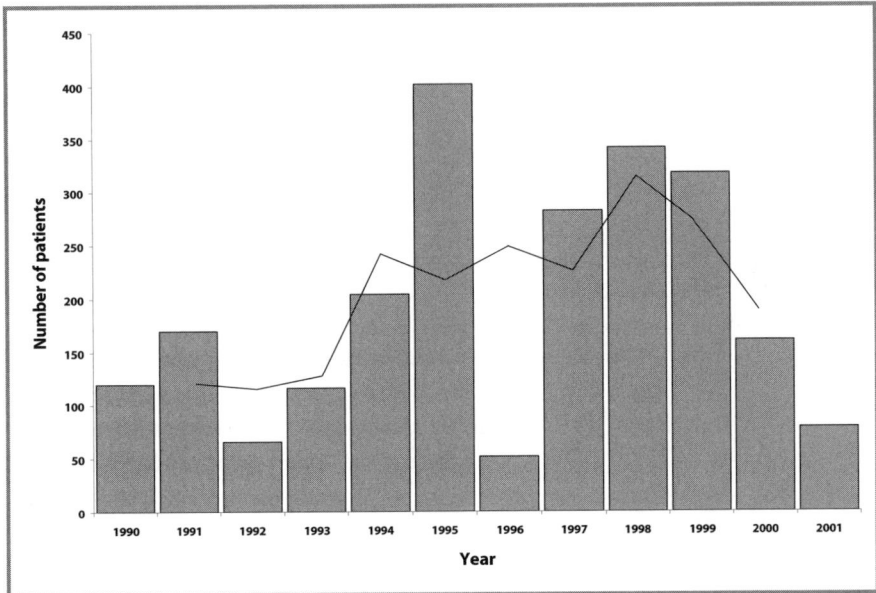

Figure 16.1: Number of E9060, emergency dog bite patients reported at the Princess Margaret Hospital, 1990–2001 (histogram), and three-year moving average (line chart).

When considering these data it should be noted that we cannot say if the bites were caused by roaming or contained, owned or unowned animals. Thus they may not necessarily be associated with changes in the number of unowned dogs or indicate that unowned dogs are more of a nuisance now than before. It should also be noted that in most cases we can expect dog bites to be caused by owned dogs.[5]

These admittance figures, which can be taken to refer to more serious dog bites, suggest that more people are now suffering from serious dog bites than in the mid-1990s. We could surmise that the increase in the more serious injuries might be associated with the rise in ownership of "image" dogs such as pit bulls. Presently, pit bulls and rottweilers[6] are the two most common breeds seen in veterinary clinics. Such dogs are associated with bites and deaths,[7] and therefore their owners need to be particularly careful if the welfare of society is to be preserved. Owned confined dogs are typically responsible for most bites,[8] but the presence of roaming dogs, such as pit bulls, threaten all society with increased risk of serious injury. The woman killed in 2001 may have been a victim of roaming pit bull types.[9]

Serious injury is one step short of death, so Figure 16.2 also shows when fatal injuries were received.[10] There are too few events to establish a pattern between the incidences of injuries and deaths, but on inspection there may be a relationship between a high number of serious injuries and death. The plateau in serious injuries after the deaths in the early nineties might have been a result of media reports calling for better control of dangerous dogs.[11] This vigilance may have gradually become lax, resulting in more serious injuries later.

Both data sets point to an underlying increase in dog bite injuries. This is a cause for concern, particularly as three citizens have been killed as a result of biting dogs.

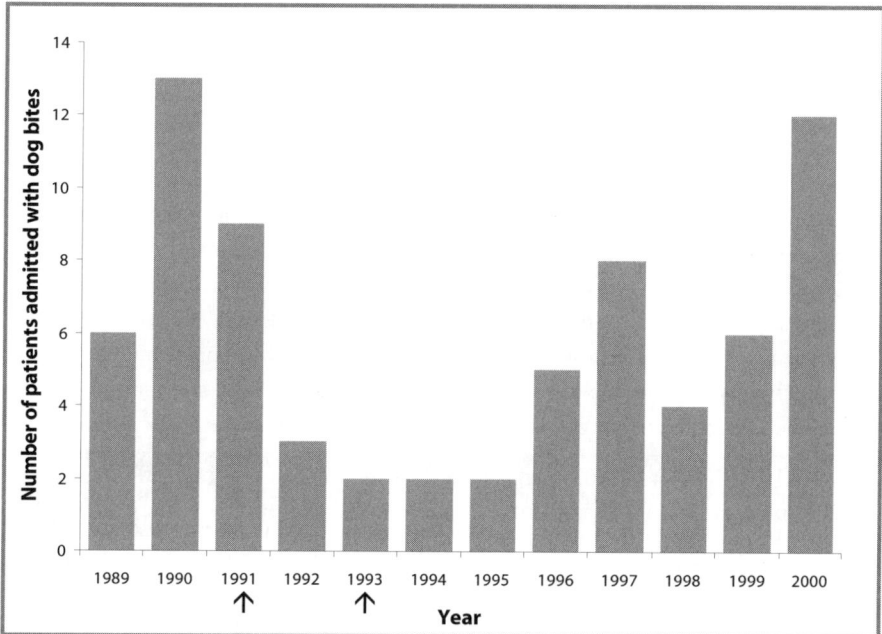

Figure 16.2: Number of admissions at the Princess Margaret Hospital due to dog bite injuries, 1989–2000. ↑ indicates fatal attacks; a third attack occurred in 2001.

Deaths due to dog attacks

As far as we have been able to find out, the first reported death due to a dog attacking a person occurred in 1991.[12] Since that time, two other people have been killed by dogs. This is a disturbing development, particularly given that the nature of the potcake, as observed since 1888 and afterwards,[13] is docile.

Since the 1980s, pit bulls and other potentially ferocious dogs (such as rottweilers) have become the image dogs of choice.[14] Although such animals would have been on the island for some years, it was only comparatively recently that they started to be commonly seen in veterinary clinics. Despite warnings from the Bahamas Humane Society about the potential risk to society posed by types such as pit bulls, there is no law about the care and breeding of these dogs.[15] Pit bulls are now the most common type of dog seen at veterinary clinics, and because of their characteristics they are favoured by companies offering guard dog services.[16]

A letter to the *Tribune* written in 1993 makes some interesting observations on the attitudes of society and government to dog attacks and to the acceptability of owning dogs capable of protecting property, even to the point of killing intruders:

> It seemed that the general opinion was that the incident was indeed regrettable [the death of an intruder by guard dogs] but that the man had no business being there. When one considers the total lack of reaction from the Attorney General's Office to this killing and to other incidents of maiming and endangerment to human life by dogs, one must assume that homicide and grievous bodily harm, by dogs are perfectly legal here. I am told that the dog responsible for the Nassau Repair yard killing also rents out at a premium: he is a now proven killer.[17]

The death in 1991 was caused by two pit bulls mauling an intruder.[18] These animals were guard-dogs protecting a business place. The second death, in 1993, was that of a nine-year-old girl who was killed by a pit bull when she visited her friend's house, in the company of the dog owner's children. The most recent death occurred in 2001, when a resident of a shared yard was killed in the middle of the night by unconfined dogs which also lived in the area. According to residents of the street in which the woman died, pit bulls were kept in the area and a Bahamas Humane Society officer considered the attack to be consistent with the work of pit bulls or pit bull types.[19] Pit bulls are allowed to roam, and have terrorized residents, so it is conceivable that roaming pit bulls, or a pit bull cross could have attacked the woman.[20] Pit bulls have also been abandoned near the airport, in the center of the island.[21] The death of the child motivated the government to refuse import licenses for pit bulls. The death caused by the unconfined dogs resulted in the killing of several potcakes in that area and the community being targeted for increased animal control efforts. As far as we know, in none of the three incidents were criminal proceedings brought against the dog owners.

The lack of sustained government action after dog attacks follows the long-standing inability of government to enforce laws and control the dog population (also mentioned in 1888) and also the unwillingness of society to effectively respond to events related to dogs, also raised in 1888. When unfortunate events occur, highlighted in the extreme by death, government officials and members of the public make calls upon each other for action, but they seem unable to unite in effective response. Although officials remind residents of their efforts to improve the situation, they also point to "irresponsible pet ownership" as a major contribution to the dog problem, but this still seems to leave society demanding that the government does "something,"[22] with some people even threatening to sue the government should they be attacked by roaming dogs, particularly pit bulls.[23] However, as shown in other countries, unless society, and in particular dog owners, recognize their responsibilities and actively participate in dog control measures, there can be no sustained or effective response, and control measures to reduce dog overpopulation may fail.[24]

Given the prolonged period over which officials and society have talked about "doing something" (at least since 1842), it is easy to get the impression that only when an even greater or spectacular disaster involving dogs and society occurs will society's demand be heard that owners are held accountable. The continuing threat of roaming dogs, such as pit bulls, has resulted in the headline "Ban pit-bulls before dogs kill a tourist!"[25] This might be interpreted (rather outrageously) to mean that the death of a tourist[26] may be worse than the death of a resident and so precipitate changes in attitudes and actions towards owners of potentially dangerous dogs.

17

What Future for the Potcake?

When we look into their [potcakes'] eyes, we see a long and painful history and also a question…'Are you the one who will love and protect me?'[1]

He [His Excellency, in 1924] thought education of the young essential in this great work [animal welfare] and better training for older ones.[2]

The old Bahamian tradition of keeping a few potcakes in the yard and feeding them table scraps, never taking them to a vet and certainly not spaying and neutering them is gradually being replaced by a new tradition of care and responsibility.[3]

There is a long history of potcakes roaming the streets of Nassau, and of tolerance towards them, despite the nuisances that they cause. We have tried to show that dog ownership—and in most cases this means potcake ownership—cannot be divorced from the cultural conditioning which surrounds the potcake. These issues give the potcake its special position in society and make it more than a mongrel. While this status may not always be favourable to potcakes, they are considered to be national icon and thus something to be preserved and nurtured. They clearly have a mild disposition and can make excellent pets and can be protective companions.

People have lived, and continue to live, more or less amicably alongside potcakes, despite disputes over territory and behaviour with humans. This long association has resulted in these animals not being perceived as a real threat to personal safety (and this perception still seems to exist even after the death of a woman by unconfined dogs) and is probably why people have not acted vigorously to constrain the dog population. The reasons for the presence of these dogs on the streets today is clear, but we may not be able to establish historically why people owned unconfined animals; was it always for protection? Our studies have shown that residents are probably as attached, if not more attached, to pets than people in other countries are. It is clear that many people have some idea as to how to look after pets even if they subscribe to common myths and misconceptions about dogs and others do not always follow their own advice. Reasons as to why owners keep their dogs outside or let them roam may appear rational to the owners, even if there are strong counter-arguments in favour of the welfare of the dogs to have them confined or keeping them inside. The reluctance of owners to neuter their dogs appears to be based on their viewing dogs in human terms and so they regard the dog's sexuality as they do their own.

It is also apparent that the welfare of the potcake has almost certainly improved since the 1850s through enactment of legislation, formation of animal welfare groups and a heightened awareness of pet care throughout much of society. Although there are some thin, sickly animals on the streets, even the roaming dogs look well-fed, and it would seem that the roaming dog of today is better fed than his ancestors. The formation of animal welfare groups, particularly in the twentieth century, has almost certainly been instrumental in increasing the welfare of the dogs and contributing to the education of owners about animal welfare.

While in theory it would appear straightforward to define the actions needed to increase dog welfare, cultural considerations must be taken into account before changes can be expected to occur.

Improvements in dog welfare typically result from more education, neutering programmes, confinement of animals, surrendering of unwanted animals and law enforcement. However, as shown above, strategies which aim to control the free-roaming dog population must accommodate the fact that the potcake is a long-standing part of Bahamian culture. For example, a neuter programme on another Bahamian island with the catchy name "Project potcake" could give the impression that its aim was to eliminate potcakes, not roaming dogs. The all too common confusion of the potcake with the roaming dog results in the impression that dog population control programmes are targeted against a Bahamian symbol. Clearly any nation would protest against a programme with such an objective.

Strategies must make clear the objectives of any population control programme, and they must be seen to be of benefit to dogs as well as owners and residents, but not having a negative impact on tourism; so while roaming dogs are undesirable, there is nothing wrong with potcakes per se. From our focus groups and surveys it is clear that non-owners have strong views about dog ownership, and so they too can influence the effectiveness of control policies. Policy makers must appreciate the difficulties that owners have in caring for their dogs and target dogs of owners that will benefit most from any intervention. Messages and actions must also take into account that male and female owners have different actions and attitudes on aspects of dog ownership.

Changes in dog ownership are likely to be slow, so sustainability of policies is of utmost importance, otherwise no long-term solution will result.[4]

Changes in pet care must start with the better-off so that "peer" pressure can be exerted throughout society and result in sustained changes in the way pets are treated. Visible policies, together with good pet ownership being practiced by public figures, can create role models which society can be expected to emulate so that society itself will expect pet care of a certain standard. The role of the better-off and leaders in society will be crucial in assisting in initiating such changes.

Successful control of the dog population cannot be expected from focusing on a single activity. Enforcement of regulations and laws may be more successful if it involved more agencies, but in a coordinated manner. Animals need to be confined, whether inside the home or behind fenced yards; if more than one animal is owned, at least all the females should be neutered. The dog license fee could be structured to provide a financial incentive to owners to neuter their dogs. Stricter penalties could also be imposed, making owners more clearly responsible for the actions of their pets, and special regulations could be applied to owners of pets that pose a threat to society. Regulations with respect to importation must be consistent with regulations on breeding within the country. All the regulations regarding dog ownership will need to be enforced if they are to have any effect; otherwise, the situation described by Powles will be repeated. Bahamians' long history of civil disobedience in paying taxes on dogs or license fees means that society will have to make considerable effort to reconsider its long-standing attitudes on dog-related taxes. In the longer term, education will institutionalize ownership practices which will ensure that the "problem" of "stray" dogs does not reoccur. These policies need to be coordinated, which requires a number of diverse organizations, both governmental (including all relevant agencies within government) and non-governmental, to cooperate with the participation of residents and communities so that their actions can effectively complement each other.[5] To ensure the sustainability of dog population control efforts, an umbrella organization may be necessary. This would encourage cooperation between all animal welfare stakeholders, which still does not always happen.[6] The importance of an integrated approach to reducing the number of dogs on the streets has been proven in other countries.[7] Funding of animal control, which has been variable and probably inadequate, needs to be addressed so that sufficient money is available to underpin the necessary long-term animal control policies.

All these policies can be implemented to control roaming dogs without being detrimental to the welfare of potcakes. As shown earlier, actions which are good for the welfare of dogs will also be good for society, as they will reduce the number of dogs which can be recruited to the roaming dog population. In fact, as the potcake population declines, as the number of unwanted dogs diminishes, the monetary value of potcakes could increase. This in turn should make them animals to be valued, like purebred dogs, and so their level of care could be expected to increase. In this way, society and potcakes will benefit.

Below we discuss components of how dog welfare could be improved within a Bahamian context.

Education

Education, in a form likely to reach all potential pet owners, is not yet available. The need for this was shown in our perception study, where almost all the respondents wanted more teaching on pet care for children. The extent of owners' knowledge about their pets was also highlighted in the neuter study. These results are in keeping with a 1974 study on classroom pets which identified a general ignorance on keeping pets, although study participants thought it would be beneficial to have pets in the classroom.[8] Television programmes on pet care can be seen in The Bahamas, *if* people choose to watch them. School "pet clubs" and summer schools offered by veterinary clinics, while excellent in themselves, must compete with other activities. Public service announcements on "responsible animal ownership," together with corporate involvement, may be ways of reaching the wider population.[9] "Walkabouts," such as those organized by cooperative groups, have been used to bring pet ownership education into communities.[10] All these methods can be employed to highlight the dog as a companionable animal and the health benefits which can accrue to dog owners.

Compulsory education at school (or through church groups[11]) is probably the only sure way of teaching potential owners about care.[12] No interviewee in our case studies had been taught pet care at school (nor are children at school today), and when a family has traditionally kept pets, practices of pet care are passed from one generation to the next and set the expectations of younger owners. Our interviews give the impression that suitable books on pet care are lacking for those who wish to learn more.[13] This suggests a need for relevant education and educational material for school children, etc., rather than what is currently available.[14] The ad hoc nature and patchy coverage of pet education currently offered by animal welfare groups has failed to have any measurable impact so far—otherwise adults would not be asking for more education on this subject and young people would be more informed on neutering than older owners. Although veterinarians should be one of the major educators on good pet ownership, many owners do not visit them, so denying the vet the opportunity to interact with owners. The current paucity of educational material for the public of all ages is a major impediment to improving the present level of pet care and knowledge of the law on animal ownership. The results of these deficiencies are vividly illustrated in our interviews. Education to alter behaviour as concerns roaming dogs and abandonment will clearly require sensitivity, particularly when it runs counter to current actions, which many people feel are acceptable, or when it appears to impinge on their liberties (such as confinement and neutering).

Although a new attempt has been initiated by animal welfare groups to place pet care in the school curriculum, this has yet to be implemented.[15] With institutional support we feel that this goal can be achieved. Education is a long-term undertaking, so even if this thrust is successful, it may be some time before its impact is seen, but this should not be seen as an impediment to this important issue. Indeed, education is probably the best long-term route to changing dog ownership practices and getting potcakes appreciated as desirable pets.

Given the influence of churches in The Bahamas,[16] teaching via churches or church groups remains an untapped opportunity, although church leaders started the first animal welfare group in Nassau. However, if some church groups have rigid views regarding animal rights, the message from the pulpit may differ from that preferred by animal welfare groups. In such cases, for the association to be effective, church leaders would need to emphasize those aspects which would benefit dogs and be in keeping with the congregation's beliefs.

While education alone need not necessarily lead to changes in behaviour or attitudes, it allows society to make more informed choices and thereby makes it aware of the result of its choices and actions.

Neutering

It is clear that all residents need to be educated on the benefits of neutering to their pets and to society. There is limited knowledge about neutering, and this, combined with owners projecting their sexuality on to that of their pets, results in relatively few animals being neutered. There appears to be little appreciation of the fact that neutering prolongs the life of dogs.

It is clear that the cost of the operation is too high for some owners, while other owners merely fail to get their pets neutered. The widespread acceptance of the general owner to neutering is reflected in the welcome given to neuter programmes in poor areas.[17] The first aim of a sustainable neuter programme should be to get richer owners to have their dogs neutered. This could then be expected to exert a downward pressure on the poorer owners to get their pets neutered. While poorer owners will always struggle to afford the cost of neutering their animals, they must become aware that it is their responsibility to at least avail their pets of the free neuter programmes which exist.

There is currently no incentive in the dog license fees to neuter a male dog, and only a $4 differential in favour of spayed females.[18] Compared with the cost of neutering, about $75, this difference is insufficient to encourage owners to neuter their animals. Increases in the license fees might result in more owners getting their dogs neutered, as it would be clear that the owner would save money by owning a neutered animal. Elsewhere, it has been shown that reduced license fees for neutered animals can indeed encourage owners to neuter their pets.[19] It has been shown that a more realistic license fee would be $20 and $31 for neutered and intact animals respectively.[20] Even these fees would be less in real terms than the fees charged in the nineteenth century. An increase in the fees might also encourage tighter enforcement of the law regarding licensing. However, the long history of non-compliance with dog taxes and the lack of enforcement means that it might be difficult to make changes in this behaviour. It should be remembered that, historically, while licenses and fines were higher than they are today, higher fees on their own do not necessarily result in compliance.

The argument that a high license fee would discourage people from licensing their dogs is, we feel, invalid, as even at the current fees few owners license their dogs. Although companionable aspects of dog ownership are considered important for single residents in some countries, our data suggest that this is not currently an important issue here. We feel that an increase in the cost of dog ownership would make owners realize that their dogs are valuable and so encourage them to look after them, even if they are "only potcakes."

Confinement

Our studies show that many owned dogs, particularly potcakes, are allowed to roam, although confining dogs is not necessarily easy, especially for those living in shared yards. However, many richer owners fail to confine their animals, and this group of people should be able to ensure that their yards are stock-proof. Confinement of dogs kept for protection needs particular emphasis, as an "off-duty" dog will provide no protection. Government policy towards low-income housing could be changed to provide fenced yards, which would assist poorer owners.

If owners knew that their roaming dogs were likely to be caught by animal control officers, this could further encourage owners to confine their animals, particularly if they had gone to the expense of having them neutered and licensed. A proactive trapping programme would also be better able to enforce the other regulations surrounding dog ownership. Education and an emphasis on the companionable aspects of dogs should help some owners to rethink their current view that it is cruel to confine dogs.

Surrendering

There appears to be resistance to surrendering unwanted animals. A change in this attitude is necessary to reduce the number of abandoned animals. Surrendering and euthanasia (death) are (we surmise) linked in the minds of owners, but attitudes on this have not yet been researched. This is also linked with the attitude of not wanting "harm" to come to dogs. Education on this matter appears to be most needed amongst the poorer people, but it is noted that even richer people abandon animals. The reluctance of owners and non-owners to surrender animals may be linked with the perception they have of humane groups. If this is so, these groups need to ensure that the public has the correct impression of their activities. Education of both owners and non-owners is required on this issue, as non-owners can also surrender animals.

The link between abandoned, owned and unowned dogs is strong, and until this link is broken, the roaming dog population will persist. Again, we feel that society has yet to grasp the importance of their role in this connection. This aspect is particularly important, as it is easy for owners to succumb to the easy option of leaving animals behind rather than surrendering them.[21]

Legislation

The current legislation is antiquated and fragmented. For example, the Dog Licence Act has not been significantly revised since 1942. Enforcement is the responsibility of independent agencies and this results in a lack of coordination and poor enforcement. For example, the police are responsible for enforcing the Penal Code Act with respect to animal cruelty, dog attacks and ferocious dogs, while the Animal Control Unit is responsible for enforcement of the Dog Licence Act and the Animal Contagious Diseases Act. New legislation is required which will increase penalties, update fees, and fill in gaps of the present laws, such as dealing with abandonment and nuisance animals.

Law enforcement

Regrettably, this country has a poor history of enforcing the law with respect to dogs. In 1803 it was clear that society was not cooperating with the tax on dog owners, and Powles, in 1888, talked of a dog license law being "abandoned." Despite subsequent laws, enforcement is still patchy. Clearly, any law, no matter how well-written, will only be of value if it is enforced. If leaders of civil society took a lead in being seen to abide by dog-related laws, they would provide useful role models and peer pressure, which should encourage others to follow.

Active enforcement of the dog licensing law would encourage owners not only to confine their animals but also to get them licensed. However, while the dog license fees are so low, there is little incentive for police to charge owners for not having bought a two-dollar license. Presently, the difficulty in establishing ownership of dogs is cited as a reason why so few cases are brought against dog owners.[22] Clearly, if dogs were licensed, ownership issues would be clearer.

While the authorities may be justified in blaming owners for "irresponsible pet ownership," they might be accused of being less than diligent in enforcing the laws they enacted, thus failing to play their part in controlling the dog population and improving animal welfare. Both the governing and governed classes have duties with respect to the law.

Reasons for dog ownership

Although many people claim to own dogs as "pets," it appears that some owners have weak bonds with their animals. It is hard to avoid the impression that dogs are primarily owned for protection, hence the animals' being kept outside. However, with the effectiveness of dogs as protectors now in question, particularly given the way many people keep their dogs, such owners need to rethink why and how they keep dogs if it is not for companionship. If the companionable aspect of dog ownership could be strengthened, other positive aspects linked with pet care should automatically follow.

With so many negative associations with potcakes current in society, it is understandable that these dogs are viewed as being "only a potcake," rather than an animal worthy of being a companion. If owners re-evaluate their relationship with their pets, this could be of benefit to both parties, although the obstacles that need to be overcome for this to happen it must be appreciated. Re-evaluation may be forced upon owners due to changes in homeownership patterns and land availability.

General

The formation of a society to protect animals in the 1890s shows how Bahamians have long recognized the need to improve the welfare of animals, and demonstrates their love and respect for them. However, the many attempts, dating back to the 1840s, to change animal welfare have been unable to produce a level of pet care which does not give cause for concern and highlights the difficulty of the goal. As has been recognized before, no one policy, or group in society, can "control the dog population." From our studies it is clear that owners, through their pet care, and in particular, abandonment and lack of confinement of dogs, contribute to the population of potcakes seen on the streets. Abandonment seems to be motivated by people having a low opinion of pot-cakes and animal welfare groups or by misguided compassion through wanting to give the unwanted dog "a chance." Lack of confinement is associated with neglect and per-ceptions that it is "cruel" to confine dogs. However, non-owners who feed animals they do not own and households that allow dogs to tip over their garbage encourage dogs into residential areas and also contribute to the nuisances which dogs cause. Law en-forcement officers who fail to enforce laws also contribute to the "stray dog problem" and passively tolerate the current actions of owners.

These actions/inactions have resulted in potcakes receiving much bad press over the years, and suggest that they are unloved or, worse, unlovable. In order for this to change, society as a whole must demand that its members, owners and non-owners, change their ways and reexamine their relationship with, and views of, potcakes. Pot-cakes should be seen as healthy, companionable pets which are truly loveable and loved by their owners. Once this happens, potcakes will become a truly positive icon of The Bahamas. Until then, it is unlikely that any great shift in their welfare will occur. Pot-cakes will continue to be blamed for the actions of their masters and when we look into a potcakes' eyes, we shall continue to see a long and painful history and also a question.

Appendix 1

Questions used in the pet attachment study

Respondents were classified by gender, age, presence of any pet, or dogs, or cats in the household.

To each question participants were asked to respond on a seven-point Likart scale from strongly disagree to strongly agree.

1. I really like seeing pets enjoy their food.
2. My pet means more to me than any of my friends (or would do if I had one).
3. I like a pet inside my own home (or would do if I had one).
4. Having pets is a waste of money.
5. House pets add happiness to my life (or would do if I had one).
6. I feel that pets should always be kept outside.
7. I spend time every day playing with my pet (or I would do if I had one).
8. I have occasionally communicated with my pet and understood what it was trying to express (or someone else's pet).
9. The world would be a better place if people would stop spending so much time caring for their pets and started caring more for other human beings instead.
10. I like to feed animals out of my hand.
11. I love pets.
12. Animals belong in the wild or in zoos, but not in the home.
13. If you keep pets in the house you can expect a lot of damage to furniture.
14. I like house pets.
15. Pets are fun but not worth the trouble of owning one.
16. I frequently talk to my pet (or would do if I had one).
17. I like animals around the home.
18. You should treat house pets with as much respect as you would a human member of your family.
19. I cry when my pet dies (or think I would if I had a pet that died).

When obtaining the attachment score, questions 4, 6, 9,1 2, and 13 were given reverse scores. The maximum score was 7 (strongly agree) and minimum 1 (strongly disagree), with 4 for "unsure."

The form was adapted from one devised by Templer.[1]

Appendix 2

Notes on the derivation of the balance sheet (Table 10.16)

It should be noted that both owned and unowned dog populations must reproduce below their potential. In the case of owned dogs this is due to many intact dogs being confined and so being unable to breed, so one pup per litter is assumed. In the case of unowned dogs, a single litter is produced, and, as many animals are sick, 1.3 pups per litter are assumed. Data from owned dogs suggest an average mortality rate of 27% per year,[1] this has been doubled for the unowned dogs, as we know they die younger than owned animals.

We know that both populations must be reasonably close to equilibrium, otherwise far more dogs would be seen on the streets. Further, other studies have shown that unowned dog populations struggle to maintain their numbers. In each case, if the number of surviving pups per litter is increased much (by even 0.5 pups per litter), both populations would increase greatly. This increase could only be offset by a major increase in adult (over 6 months) mortality.

Other calculations show that food is a limiting factor in the increase of dogs that are fed handouts,[2] although this does not prevent modest increases in population. Thus, both dog populations are probably limited by food availability, and hence by the growth in the number of households. The number of households is projected by the Department of Statistics, to increase by 14% in the next 10 years, so the dog populations could also increase by a similar percentage.

Owned dogs

The opening balance is obtained directly from the number of dogs people claim to own per household. The high death rate among owned dogs is due to lack of adequate pet care; about two-thirds of all owned dogs see the vet less than once a year. Most owned dogs are intact, so dogs which roam can breed with other free-roaming dogs.

A large number of unwanted animals may be transferred from the owned to unowned population.[3] Although this number may not appear to represent a large fraction of the owned population (10%), it is crucial in sustaining the unowned population and could represent about 65% of this population. Increased neutering would reduce the number of unwanted dogs and consequently the number abandoned.

Dogs that are removed illegally[4] may compensate for the number of dogs imported, which of course increases the population. A conservative estimate has been used for the number of imported dogs. Imports could be between 2–5% of the current owned dog population.[5]

Unowned dogs

The opening balance for the unowned population is estimated from the percentage of households which feed dogs they do not own (assuming one unique dog per household) minus the 28% of owned dogs which roam. The total roaming dog population would be estimated at about 32,000. Disease (exhibited by a low life expectancy) is expected to be the limiting factor on the unowned population. Food is not currently a limiting factor[6] (Fielding, unpublished); however, food could expect to limit the growth of the population beyond 2% per year.

Notes

Chapter 1: New Providence

1. Culmer, J. (ed.) (1948). *Letters from the Bahama Islands*. Written in 1823–4. Letter III, p. 11. Second edition. The Providence Press, Nassau.

2. Department of Statistics (2002). *Report of the 2000 census of population & housing*. Ministry of Economic Development, Nassau.

3. *Bahamas Handbook 2001* (2000). Etienne Dupuch Jr. Publications, Nassau.

4. And also that of the Turks and Caicos Islands.

5. Albury, P. (1975). *The story of the Bahamas*. Macmillan Education Ltd., London.

6. Craton, M. (1986). *A history of The Bahamas*. San Salvador Press, Canada. 3rd edition.

7. For more on this topic see Williams, P. M. (1996). Ethnic minorities in The Bahamas. *Journal of the Bahamas Historical Society* 18: 12–20.

8. Craton, M. (1986). Op. cit.

9. Department of Statistics, (2002). *Report of the 2000 Census of population and housing*. Ministry of Economic Development, Nassau.

10. *Report of the 2000 Census of population and housing*. Op. cit.

11. Craton, M. and Saunders G. (1998). *Islanders in the stream. A history of The Bahamian people*. Volume II. University of Georgia Press, Athens.

12. Craton, M. and Saunders G. (1992). *Islanders in the stream. A history of The Bahamian people*. Volume I. University of Georgia Press, Athens. And Craton, M. and Saunders G. (1998). Op. cit.

13. Bahamas Handbook 2001. Op. cit.

14. Bahamas Handbook 2001. Op. cit.

15. Bahamas Handbook 2001. Op. cit.

16. Department of Statistics (2001). 2002 Department of Statistics, The Commonwealth of The Bahamas. Department of Statistics, Nassau. It should be noted that for practical purposes that one Bahamian dollar is equivalent to one United States dollar.

17. ". . . two tourists had to beat a retreat after being accosted by a boisterous pack of stray potcakes. . . . What was really disturbing about this incident was . . . the reaction of the Bahamian vendors and patrons. . . . Patrons continued their loud banter as though the tourists and the dogs didn't exist." The Tribune (2002). Let's grow out of this backward Potcake culture. 18 February, p. 5.

18. The Tribune (2002). Jet ski operators attract negative tourism publicity. 9 April, p. 1B.

19. Rolle, L. (1998). Personal communication, Ministry of Housing, Nassau.

20. Lawlor, A. (2002). Personal communication, School of English, The College of the Bahamas.

Chapter 2: Dogs in New Providence

1. The Nassau Guardian (2001). Editorial: The stray dogs problem. 11 May, p. 8A.

2. Albury, P. (1975). *The story of The Bahamas.* Macmillan Caribbean.

3. Northcroft, G. J. H. (1900). *Sketches of Summerland.* The Nassau Guardian, Nassau.

4. It is conjectured that two of the primary reasons man took dogs into his home were food (Coppinger, R. and Coppinger, L. (2001). *Dogs: A startling new understanding of canine origin, behavior, and Evolution.* Scribner, New York), and companionship (Levinson, B. M. (1969). Pet-orientated child psychotherapy. Charles C. Thomas, Springfield IL.)

5. Northcroft, G. J. H. (1900). Op. cit. Quoting Juan La Costa.

6. Northcroft, G. J. H. (1900). Op. cit.

7. Lightbourn, M. E. (2001). The primeval forest—revisited. *Bahamas Journal of Science* 8(2): 13–21.

8. These first colonists of New Providence arrived between 1648 and 1666. Eleutherian Adventurers brought "stock" animals to The Bahamas, which may have included dogs; Craton, M. and Saunders G. (1992). *Islanders in the stream. A history of The Bahamian people.* Volume I. University of Georgia Press, Athens. As far as we are aware, no archaeological evidence of dogs from the time of the Lucayans have been found; Personal communication by Buckner, S. (2003). Nor have excavations of plantation areas of the 1820s found evidence of dogs; see Farnsworth, P. (1994). Archaeological excavations at Promised Land Plantation, New Providence. *Journal of the Bahamas Historical Society* 18: 33–42.

9. Coren, S. (2002). *The pawprints of history.* The Free Press, New York. The use of dogs as aggressors was revisited in the 1790s when it was suggested that dogs be used to capture fugitive slaves. Reported in Ingram, K. E. (1975). *Manuscripts relating to Commonwealth Caribbean countries in United States and Canadian Repositories.* Caribbean University Press & Bowker Publishing Company: UK.

10. Albury, P. (1975). Op. cit. Picture of "Woodes Rogers and family at Fort Nassau," facing p. 134, belonging to Lady Virginia Christie. This picture suggests that the upper classes owned dogs and that they were of sufficient importance to the owners be included in their portraits.

11. More recent pictures which have dogs include Eddie Minnis' 1976 picture of Dean's Lane and others. (For example, see http://www.bahamas.mall.bs/art/minnis/eddie2.htm#Eddie. Several potcakes are included in a picture by Melissa Maura (1983). There is also a series of prints by Leo Brown which include roaming dogs. E.g.: The Bahamian Village (1998) and Dwelling Places (1999). A greeting card published by *web & tomland* depicts two dogs chewing a woman's skirt in a painting by Amos Ferguson. In 2000, the 70-cent postage stamp issued to highlight the work of the Bahamas Humane Society featured potcakes. A series of generic "Caribbean" pictures for tea trays etc., by G. Gobinet, includes one which features a large number of roaming dogs. This points to roaming dogs as being a feature of the wider Caribbean landscape.

12. Feduccia. A. (Ed.) (1985). *Catesby's birds of Colonial America.* University of North Carolina Press, Chapel Hill, p. 168.

13. This is its current name. It is also called Dog Flea Lane on some maps. Mather, J. and Fielding, W. J. (2001). The threat posed to personal health by dogs in New Providence. *Bahamas Journal of Science* 8(2): 39–45.

14. Bruce, P. (1782). *Bahamian interlude. Being an account of the life at Nassau in the Bahama Islands in the eighteenth century, reported from the "Memoirs of Peter Henry Bruce Esq.," published in London in 1782.* Reprinted 1949, John Culmer Ltd., London.

15. *Votes of the House of Assembly* (1803). 22 November 1802. Robert Wilson, Nassau.

16. *Votes of the House of Assembly* (1804). 26 November 1803. Robert Wilson, Nassau.

17. Culmer, J. (ed.) (1948). *Letters from the Bahama Islands.* Written in 1823–4. Letter XIII, p. 71. Second edition. The Providence Press, Nassau.

18. This observation contrasts with the complaint from an English tourist in 1970 who bemoaned the barking at night, "what masses of dogs Nassau seems to have." The Nassau Guardian (1970). Letter to the editor. 28 January, p. 4.

19. McQueen, N. (1830). *The Bahama almanac and register for the year 1830.* "Compiled, printed and sold by Neil McQueen," Nassau, p. 43. Values have been converted to present values assuming a current exchange rate of £1=US$1.60 and the historical value of sterling from McCusker, J. J. (2001). Comparing the purchasing power of money in Great Britain from 1264 to any other year including the present. Economic History Services. http://www.eh.net/hmit/ppowerbp/

20. At that time these landmarks could be regarded as being the boundaries of the upper-class district of Nassau.

21. Johnson, H. (1996). *The Bahamas from slavery to servitude 1783–1933.* University Press of Florida.

22. Royal Gazette (1837). Lost or stolen. 11 January, p. 3.

23. Anderson, G. C. (1843). An Act for imposing a tax on dogs, 1841. *Laws of The Bahamas in force on the 14 March 1842.* "Printed at the office of 'The Observer'," Nassau.

24. Craton, M. and Saunders G. (1992). Grant's Town (started from 1825) was an extension of Negro Town. Op. cit. Slavery was fully abolished in 1834; full emancipation came in 1838 after the ex-slaves had served a four-year apprenticeship.

25. Johnson, H. (1996). Op. cit.

26. Officer, L.H. (2002). Exchange rate between the United States dollar and forty other countries 1913–1999. Economic History Services, E.H. Net. http://www.eh.net/hmit/exchangerates.

27. The Nassau Guardian (1849). Convictions, &c. 8 September, p. 1.

28. Malcolm, O. D. (1901). *The Statute law of The Bahamas, comprising all acts of the General Assembly of The Bahama Islands in force to 62 Victoria, Chapter 33. inclusive.* Eyre and Spottiswoode.

29. Moseley, E. C. (1876). *An almanac for 1876, with a history of the Bahamas.* "Compiled, printed and published by Edwin Charles Moseley," Nassau, p. 50.

30. Beck, A. (1973). *The ecology of stray dogs. A study of free-ranging urban animals.* Purdue University Press, reprinted 2002.

31. Malcolm, O. D. (1901). An Act to impose a tax on dogs, and for other purposes, 1856. Op. cit.

32. Albury, P. (1975). Op. cit. Picture of "Unloading cotton at Nassau," centre page (this picture, from the *Illustrated London News*, April 18, 1864, suggests that roaming dogs were present in public places by the mid-1800s); The London Illustrated News (1864). 10 December.

33. The Nassau Guardian (1863). December 5, p. 3.

34. Malcolm, O. D. (1901). An Act to amend the Statute Law of The Bahama islands relative to larceny and other offences connected therewith, 1865. Op. cit.

35. "And here is a man with a dog, grumbling because he has to pay duty on him." Drysdale, W. (1885). *In sunny lands: Out-door life in Nassau and Cuba.* Harper & Brothers, New York; Moseley, E. C. (1879). *An almanac for 1879, with a history of the Bahamas.* "Compiled, printed and published by Edwin Charles Moseley," Nassau, p. 47.

36. Ives, C. (1880). *The isles of summer. Nassau and The Bahamas.* The author, New Haven, Connecticut, p. 125.

37. Ives, *op. cit*, p. 126.

38. Drysdale, W. (1885). Op. cit.

39. Drysdale, W. (1885). Op. cit.

40. Malcolm, O. D. (1901). An Act to consolidate the laws relating to police regulations, 1873. Op. cit.

41. Quoted from Drysdale's book. Drysdale, W. (1885). Op. cit.

42. Powles, L. D. (1888). *The land of the pink pearl. Recollections of life in The Bahamas.* Reprinted 1996, Media Publishing Ltd., Nassau, pp. 76–77.

43. "'Couldn't get much dog's meat to-day, sir'" and ". . . unhappy man who tries to keep a big dog fat in Nassau!" when referring to the cost of dog food. Drysdale, W. (1885). Op. cit.

44. The Nassau Guardian (1892). Editorial. 26 October, p. 2.

45. The Nassau Guardian (1898). May 11, p. 2.

46. The Nassau Guardian (1898). The dog, the man, and the meat. 16 April, p. 1.

47. Northcroft (1900). Op. cit.

48. Johnstone, W. K. (1973). *Poems and prose with photographs of old Nassau.* Brice Publishing Co. Ltd., Nassau.

49. For example: Anon (undated). Framed photograph in the Department of Archives entitled "Liberated African settlement," picture No. 22 and Anon (1982), Settlements in New Providence PRO/5/10 Album #2.

50. Anon (2003). *Junkanoo & religion. Christianity and cultural identity in The Bahamas.* Papers presented at the Junkanoo symposium, March 2002. Media Publishing, Nassau; Eneas, C. W. (1976). *Bain Town.* Privately published by Cleveland & Muriel Eneas, Nassau, Bahamas.

51. "Obe" is known today as "Obeah." See McCartney, T. (1976). *Ten, ten, the Bible ten – Obeah in The Bahamas.* Timpaul Publishers Co., Nassau.

52. Reported in: Williams, J. J. (1932). *Voodoos and obeahs. Phases of West India witchcraft.* AMS Press, New York. Reprinted 1970.

53. Williams, J. J. (1932). Op. cit.; McCartney, T. (1976). Op. cit.

54. Malcolm, O. D. (1901). An act to consolidate the duties on imports . . . 1895. Op. cit.; Government of The Bahamas (1987). (ed. Bryce, G.) *Subsidiary legislation of the Bahamas.* BPPC Wheaton Ltd., Exeter, UK. Chapter 345.

55. Northcroft (1900). Op. cit.; The Nassau Guardian (1942). House of Assembly. 17 February, p. 2.

56. Mosley, M. (1942). *Bahamas acts passed in the year 1942.* Nassau Guardian, Nassau.

57. Roberts, E. D. (1991). Aspects of life in Nassau and The Bahamas during the 1940s and 1950s. *Journal of the Bahamas Historical Society,* 13(1), 18–23.

58. Government of the Commonwealth of The Bahamas (2002). Act No.1 of 2002 Minimum wages *The Statute Law of The Bahamas 1799–2002 in force on the 2nd April 2002.* Juta & Co, Ltd.

59. The Nassau Guardian (1942). What do you think? 17 February, p. 2.

60. For example: The Nassau Guardian (2003). Stray dogs threaten tourism, Wilchcombe says. 30 January, pp. 1A, 11A.

61. The Nassau Guardian (1943). Where is the dog catcher? 6 September, p. 2.

62. The Nassau Guardian (1944). Editorial: Stray dog nuisance. 31 January, p. 2.

63. The Nassau Guardian (1965). Letter to the editor, 3 February, p. 6.

64. The Nassau Guardian (1943). Home for dog wanted. 13 September, p. 2.

65. The Tribune (1932). Bahamas Humane Society report for last week. February 25, p. 1; and The Nassau Guardian (1932). Activities of the Bahamas Humane Society. 24 February, p. 4.

66. The Nassau Guardian (1944). Editorial: Stray dog nuisance, 31 January, p. 2, reports that 112 dogs were caught last month and 727 caught in 1943. The Nassau Guardian (1944). Editorial: The stray dog nuisance. 24 February, p. 2, reports on dogs in Parliament Street. On more recent reports, see, for example, a picture of a roaming dog near the House of Assembly, The Tribune (1999). Stray dogs: A complicated problem. 25 February, p. 10. Samuels, D. (2003). Personal communication, reports that dogs still roam on Montague Beach.

67. For example, letters to The Tribune, 1950, 5 April 5; 1968, 11 January, p. 3, 1975, 3 January, p. 3 as well as other references cited by us.

68. The Tribune (1999). Stray dogs: A complicated problem. 25 February, p. 10.

69. The Punch (2002). All animals deserve your kindness if hit by vehicle. 15 August, p. 19.

70. Between 1992 and 1996, crimes against property increased by 22% and crime against persons by 25%. Department of Statistics (1999). *Statistical abstract 1999.* Ministry of Economic Development, Nassau.

71. The Guardian (2001). Editorial: The stray dogs problem. 11 May, p. 8A.

72. For example: The Nassau Guardian (2002). Letter to editor, 3 October, p. 8A.

73. The Nassau Guardian (1998). Stray dogs seen as 'a people's problem' 8 May, pp. 11A, 15A.

74. The Tribune (2003). Letter to the editor. 13 August, p. 4.

75. The Tribune (2001). Minister: we're tackling dog issue but public must help. 19 September, p. 6.

76. The Nassau Guardian (2003). Dog act to be reviewed. 27 January, p. 11; The Tribune (2003). Tourist dog attack 'could have been avoided'. 30 January, pp. 1, 11;The Nassau Guardian (2003). Editorial. 27 January, p. 10.

77. Turnquest, S. (2000). Personal communication. See Chapter 10.

78. The Nassau Guardian (1997). Vicious pit bulls upset family. 29 April, pp. 1A, 3A.

79. The Tribune (2001). Pitbull infiltration 'making our potcakes turn vicious'. 4 October, p. 8. Willis, M. B. (1995). Genetic aspects of dog behaviour with particular reference to working ability. In: *The domestic dog: its evolution, behaviour and interactions with people*. (ed. Serpell, J.). Cambridge University Press, pp. 52–64.

80. For example, negative publicity followed the fatal mauling of a woman in 2001. The Tribune (2000). Ongoing plan to keep out rabies. 9 May, p. 5. So far, there has been no confirmed case of West Nile Virus (The Nassau Guardian (2003) West Nile case feared, 8 August, pp. 1A, 5A) or Monkey pox in The Bahamas.

81. As reported by all the clinics in our 1998/99 census.

82. The disease could enter the country via other vectors, see above report.

83. For example: The Tribune (2001). Our pets were deliberately poisoned, say dog owners. 29 October, p. 3.

84. Hubrecht, R. (1995). The welfare of dogs in human care. In: *The domestic dog: its evolution, behaviour and interactions with people*. Ed. Serpell, J., pp. 179–198. Cambridge University Press.

85. The Nassau Guardian (1924). Editorial: History repeating itself. 11 December, p. 2. This law made it unlawful to allow cows to roam or to allow dogs to intimidate others. For example: The Nassau Guardian (1849). 12 May, p. 1; and 8 September, p. 1.

86. Anderson, G. C. (1843). Malicious injuries to property, 1841. *Laws of The Bahamas in force on the 14 March 1842.* "Printed at the office of 'The Observer'," Nassau. Laws regarding animal cruelty are currently included in the Penal Code, and it is the responsibility of the police to enforce them.

87. The Nassau Guardian (1892). Editorial. 26 October, p. 2; and The Nassau Guardian (1892). Letter to the editor, 24 September, p. 2.

88. For example: The Nassau Guardian (1892). Letter to the editor. 1 October, p. 2.

89. The Nassau Guardian (1924). Op. cit.

90. For example: The Nassau Guardian (2001). Animal rights activist wants BGI stray animals neutered. 10 May, p. 12A.

91. The Nassau Guardian (1974). 'Animal week' offers opportunity and challenge. 16 November, p. 6.

92. On the stray dog issue, see our perception study below. Nassau itself is commonly re-garded as "central," and the other areas are described in relation to Nassau. As Nassau lies on the north coast of the island, no one lives "north."

93. Based upon the household income by area in our 1998 study.

94. The Nassau Guardian (1998). Letter to the editor: Stray dogs not restricted to Over The Hill. 4 June, p. 2A. On the social/economic aspect, see the results from our perception study in Chapter 13.

95. Saunders, T. and Storr, D. (2002). Roaming dogs. Unpublished research project for Course 421, Man and the Environment, The College of The Bahamas.

Chapter 3: Potcakes

1. The Tribune (2000). Packs of wild dogs pose major problem. 20 November, p. 3.

2. "Pot cake" was in use in the early 1920s with regard to cooked rice and peas, *"which some of us children liked."* Eneas, C. W. (1976). *Bain Town.* Cleveland & Muriel Eneas, Nas-sau, Bahamas, p. 64.

3. First two definitions from Holon, J. A. and Shilling, A. W. (1982). *Dictionary of Bahamian English.* Lexik House Publishers, New York; third definition from Allsopp, R. (1996). *Dictionary of Caribbean English usage.* Oxford University Press.

4. Only in The Bahamas and Turks and Caicos are mixed breed dogs called potcakes. A dis-tinction is sometimes made on documentation associated with the importation of mongrel dogs; on the American export documents the animals can be described as of "mixed" breed, while on The Bahamian import permit they are re-classified as "pot-cake."

5. The Bahamas and the Turks and Caicos Islands share a common history which may ex-plain this common usage. "In 1776, after being controlled by the Spanish, French and British, Turks and Caicos became part of the Bahamas colony, but attempts to integrate failed and were abandoned in 1848." http://www.geographia.com/turks-caicos/general/history/. See also Williams, P.M. (1989). The separation of The Turks and Caicos is-lands from The Bahamas. *Journal of the Bahamas Historical Society.* 11(1): 12–15. On the "Potcake Foundation" in Turks and Caicos, see http://potcake0.tripod.com/pg1.htm.

6. We have failed to find "potcake" or "pot cake" in on-line dictionaries (e.g.: American Heritage Dictionary) or in: Ayto, J. (1998). *The Oxford Dictionary of Slang.* Oxford University Press, Oxford, UK, or *The Shorter Oxford English Dictionary* (1973). Op. cit.

7. It is also just possible that "potcake" is a corruption of an African (Yoruba?) word; but this has yet to be investigated. In the 1870s, African languages were still spoken in Nassau. Moseley, E. C. (1876). *An almanac for 1876, with a history of the Bahamas.* "Compiled, printed and published by Edwin Charles Moseley," Nassau, p. 70. Even in the 1920s, African patois was still spoken in Bain Town, a settlement (once) to the south of Nas-sau. Eneas, C. W. (1976). *Bain Town.* Privately published by: Cleveland & Muriel Eneas, Nassau, Bahamas, p. 62.

8. Allsopp, R. (1996). *Dictionary of Caribbean English usage.* Oxford University Press. This dictionary suggests that potcakes were fed rice and grits. The dictionary also indicates

that dogs in Guyana are called "Rice dogs" which are "worthless as a watch dog." See later observations about the watch dog abilities of potcakes.

9. One (extreme?) definition of "truly Bahamian" is a person who "of necessity has eaten potcake." The Guardian (2001). Letter to the editor, 1 November. http://www. bahamainfo.com/news_display.php?prid=2306&src=nassau. It is worth noting that the dictionary definition does not consider potcake as something which needs to be unpleasant to eat or a poor person's food, which seems to contradict the impression given by the letter writer. In fact, some people consider potcake to be a delicacy.

10. Veenkamp, B. (2002), Winning the dog wars. Times of the islands. The international magazine of the Turks & Caicos. Spring: 27–31.

11. Thorne, J. (1995). Feeding behaviour of domestic dogs and the role of experience. In: *The domestic dog: its evolution, behaviour and interactions with people.* Ed. Serpell, J.: 103–114. Cambridge University Press.

12. In 2002, JM's aunt, 86-year old Dorothea Brown, claimed she recalled her grandparents calling dogs potcakes. She thinks that slaves or ex-slaves coined the name. If this is so, the name potcake would have been used when Powles was writing. Given his interest in the non-white population, it is curious that he failed to say that this was the name it used for dogs. In a 1943 report in The Nassau Guardian (6 September, p. 3) the word "cur" is used. (It is worth noting the definition given in the *Shorter Oxford Dictionary* (1973), Little, W., Fowler, H.W., Coulson, J. (rev. and ed. by Onions, C. T.; 3rd edition rev. by Friedrichsen, G. W. S.). Oxford University Press, Oxford, of cur: "(1) a dog: now always depreciative; a low bred or snappish dog. (2) A surly, ill-bred, or cowardly fellow.") Brenda Lynes, a housewife aged 82 in 2003, has "always" used the word "potcake" for dog, but she did not know the meaning of the word "cur." This might suggest that the term "cur" was used in the press in preference to "potcake," which was, until recently, considered too close to slang to be used in respectable newspapers. In 1965, Sir Stafford Sands refers to a "stray dog" as just a "tan mongrel." The Nassau Guardian (1965). Letter to the editor, 30–31 January, p. 4. Another explanation for the current use of the word potcake is given by (amongst others) Winston Ferguson, living in Grand Bahama in 2002. He was born in 1935, and claims that the use of the word potcake did not commonly occur until about the 1960s, when pure-bred dogs were imported. Potcake was then used to distinguish between local and imported (breed) dogs.

13. The Nassau Guardian (1970). Girls give new look to Humane Society. 30 April, Section B p. 2.

14. Balfe, P. (2002). Personal communication. Balfe arrived in the Bahamas in 1964, and recalls using the word on health certificates from at least 1969. Then, he says, potcakes from different islands had different characteristics which he could identify. Since the 1980s, he has seen fewer "pure potcakes" and more "potcake crosses." This suggests that the "classic" potcake may now be rare, at least in New Providence.

15. Anon (1973). The obeah woman. Nassau Guardian Weekend Magazine. 13 May, p. 6. It is not clear if the short story is new or repeats one from 1952.

16. The Nassau Guardian (1960). When is a cur not a cur? 8 March, pp. 1, 11.

17. As we note later, the term "breed" is not strictly interpreted as pedigree, but rather "recognisably." The dictionary's definition may be the result of the Bahamas Kennel Club setting a "standard" for potcakes.

18. These students were in two classes with median ages of 17 and 18 years old and predominantly female. September 2002.

19. Kerr. J. (undated). Potcakes. The great dogs of the Abaco islands. Abaco Life. http://go-abacos.com/news/ablife/news_life_contd2.html.

20. Bahamas Kennel Club (undated). The Bahamian potcake standard (Subject to change). Bahamas Kennel Club, Nassau.

21. The Nassau Guardian (1974). Picture caption, "…purebred potcake was second runner-up…" in a dog show. 18 February, p. 1.

22. What's On. The ultimate on-line guide to The Bahamas (1999).The Royal Bahamian potcake. 1 August. http://www.whatsonbahamas.com.

23. Beck, A. (2002). Personal communication.

24. Paraphrased from Stubbs' "The cry of the potcake."

25. The Nassau Guardian (2002). The stone that the builder rejected. 14 March, http://www.bahamainfo.com/news_display.php?prid=4409&src=nassau

26. The former expression from MORE94FM (1998). Guest on the Steve McKinney Show, 2 October (Radio programme); the latter from The Tribune (2002). Let's grow out of this backward Potcake culture. 18 February, p. 5.

27. Potcakes are not bought or sold. If it happens, it would be most rare.

28. The Nassau Guardian (2002). Op. cit.

29. Definition provided by students in psychology at The College of The Bahamas, September 2002.

30. Potcake (2002). No title. 25 November. http://onebahamas.com/Potcake. Accessed 5 June 2003.

31. For example: Cover to the LP/tape "Der real ting!!" (1976). Luck Enterprises, Nassau.

32. Minnis, E. (2002). Personal communication.

33. For example: The Tribune (1978). 9 May, p. 4.

34. See Minnis' web page, http://eddieminnis/com.

35. Minnis, E. (2002). Personal communication.

36. Prior to these songs, there appear to have been no songs about potcakes, not even during the "Golden age" of Bahamian music. Munnings, F. (2003). Musician, personal communication.

37. Minnis, E. (2000). "Mix-up dog." http://eddieminnis/com/Mix-up-dog.htlm. Note that even in this context the potcake is seen as being promiscuous.

38. The Tribune (2003). Bishop: I won't apologize. Religious leader stands by "gay" remarks. 15 July, pp. 1, 11.

39. The CD is undated. Distributed by Down Home Productions Inc, Freeport Grand Bahama.

40. From the CD *Combina Time* (2002). www.cdbaby.com/cd/loveyforbes4.

41. Traditionally the dog is the symbol of loyalty, and this chorus suggests a one-sided loyalty.

42. This concern reflects that of Bahamian youth; while 89% of 11–12 year olds thought that their mother cared "a lot" for them, this decreased to 80% by the time they were 16 or over. The corresponding figures for fathers were 71% and 53%. Health Information Unit (2001). Bahamas youth health survey. Ministry of Health. Unpublished.

43. Rotary and AWARE have both used this song in their activities.

44. For example: "Gods and spirits are summoned through the portal divine" by Ian Strachan. Caribbean writer on line poetry, University of Virgin Islands, 23 July 2001. http://www.thecaribbeanwriter.com/volume14/v14p10.html. Accessed 5 June 2003.

45. These associations go beyond that merely of women calling a man a "dog" or "no good," who has offended them (The Tribune (2002). Set the standard. 16 January, p. C1) as these are used in other countries.

46. In the office in which JM's relation worked, the song was taken to refer to human relationships, rather than a song about potcakes.

47. From a page on advice on adult relations:
    ". . . should I continue the casual relationship . . . ?" Reply: "What are you, a potcake, willing to accept any scrap of meat that's thrown your way?" The Confidential Source (2002). Letter to Roach on Ya bread! 28, 22 May, p. 5.

48. Moss, P. A. (1974). Development of family life: challenge to the church in The Bahamas. M.A. Thesis. St. John's University, Collegeville, Minnesota. It has been found that 31% of households are headed by females, with no male present. Department of Statistics (2002). *Report of the 2000 census of population and housing.* Ministry of Economic Development, Nassau. Also 47% of school children do not have their father living at home. Health Information Unit (2001). Op. cit. Sweet-hearting occurs when men, sometimes married, have one or more mistresses whom they may also support. The Tribune (2002). Sweetheart trap. 14 August, p. 1C.

49. Brennen, B. H. (1999). A new breed of Bahamian men needed. Sounds of encouragement. www.tagnet.org/encouragement/newmenneeded.htm.

50. Warning, this is an adult website: Dr_ Yellow daily links 100% FREE eye candy raw smut. dryellow.com/index25.html.

51. This quotation from The Guardian (2002) came from an article on religion, thus making this reference of interest as the writer seems to make a subconscious reference to the potcake's sexuality by using the word "prowess."

52. The Confidential Source (2003). Cartoon. 19 February, p. 14; The Tribune (2003). Picture caption "It's a dog's life." 16 May, p. 12.

53. The Tribune (2001). Embassy "will reach out to all – pledge," 7 December, p. 10.

54. For example: Rotary Club Nassau Sunrise Special Supplement (2002). Who let the dogs out? March, p. 14. Published by The Tribune.

55. Brennen, B. H. (1999). When parents nurture, children blossom. Sounds of encouragement. www.tagnet.org/encouragement/whenparentsnurture.htm.

56. The Punch (2002). A woman with two dogs and a Kemp Road gallery. 12 December, p. 28.

57. JM has personally assisted tourists in having potcakes exported to their homelands; and see The Tribune (1999), 9 February, p. 8C. Statistic from our perception study in New Providence; see Chapter 8.

58. The Bahama Journal (2003). Potcake dogs finding love in foreign homes. 12 August. http://www.jonescommunicationsltd.com/journal/index.php?url_channel_id=0&url_s ubchannel_id_&url_publish_channel_id=159&well_id=2

59. For example: At the souvenir shop at Traveller's Rest, West Bay Street.

60. Newton, S. (2003). "They call me potcake...." The dilemma of The Bahamian mongrel. What's on. The complete guide to Nassau & Paradise Island. May, p. 15.

61. This ambivalence is also noted in the responses in our perception study.

62. Descriptions from The Tribune (2002). Potcake to put the bite on drugs. 19 November, p. 7; and What's on. The Ultimate on-line guide to The Bahamas. (2002). Dispelling the pot cake myth. 30 June. http://www.whatsonbahamas.com.

63. *"No-one listens to a poor man's wisdom,"* said Bertram Mills. The Tribune (2002). MP Declarations 'farce'. 16 April, pp. 1, 11.

64. The Tribune (2001). Letter to the editor: Pitbulls must be banned to stop deaths. 26 September, p. 4.

65. Beetz, A. (2002). Love, violence and sexuality in relationships between humans and animals. PhD thesis. Friedrich-Alexander Universität Erlangen-Nürnberg.

66. The Tribune (2000). A man called potcake. 2 October, p. 9.

67. The Tribune (2002). Mascot takes anti-drug campaign to schools. 11 January, p. 7; The Tribune (2002). Potcake to put the bite on drugs. 19 November, p. 7; The Tribune (2001). Students urged: don't give pets a dog's life. 6 December, p. 14.

68. Lightbourn, C. (1989). Weekly episodes in "Youth Beat," *Tribune,* 3 June–22 July.

69. Bain, A. (2003). *Ninety-nine potcakes.* Macmilllan Caribbean, Oxford, UK.

70. See www.biminilove.org/potcake.html; and Welcome Bahamas. Op. cit.

71. Although the Bahamas Kennel Club has a section for potcakes in their dog shows, there are few entries. At the 2003 dog show there were only three listed entries for the potcake class. Programme for Bahamas Kennel Club 22nd International all breed dog show and obedience trials 15–16 March 2003.

72. Welcome Bahamas (1998/99). True true Bahamians. Potcakes, a unique breed. Etienne Dupuch Jr. Publishers, Nassau. Pp. 38, 39.

73. "Life's hard when you're a potcake, running round the streets all day, barking at passing cars, rummaging through bin-bags and scratching off those pesky dog fleas. By the time the noonday sun is at its height, even the perkiest potcake feels dog tired. This flat-out family of five were sharing some much-needed shade on the roadside as cars passed by only inches from their noses and feet in East Bay Street." The Tribune (2002). We're just dog tired. 17 August 2002, p. 10. Or The Tribune (2003). This is our beach! 9 April, p. 1.

74. Serpell, J. (1995). From paragon to pariah: some reflections on human attitudes to dogs. In: *The domestic dog: its evolution, behaviour and interactions with people.* Ed. Serpell, J.: 179–198. Cambridge University Press.

75. The Tribune (2001). Attacks by stray dogs: MP calls for new controls. 18 September, p. 5.

76. Aspects of animal symbols and Jungian psychology are discussed by Beetz, A. (2002). Op. cit.

77. This is discussed further in our section on neutering.

78. The concept of "cultural competence" discussed in a slightly different context also applies here. Kaufmann, M. E. (1999). *The relevance of cultural competence to the link between violence to animals and people.* In child abuse, domestic violence, and animal abuse. Ascione, F. R. and Arkow, P. (eds.). Purdue University Press, West Lafayette, Indiana, 260–270.

Chapter 4: Organizations Associated with Dogs

1. The Nassau Guardian (2001). Animal Care. September 18. http://www.bahamainfo.com/news_display.php?prid=1409&src=nassau.

2. More information about the Bahamas Humane Society can be found at http://www.bahamashumanesociety.com/index.php.

3. The term "shelter" is not used in The Bahamas. The Bahamas Humane Society is the only organisation in New Providence that would be termed a shelter in America.

4. For example: The Tribune (2002). Pet of the week. 25 May, p. 9.

5. Government of The Bahamas (1987). (Ed. Bryce, G.) *Statute law of the Bahamas 1799–1987.* A. Wheaton & Co. Ltd., Exeter, UK. Chapter 77.

6. Bahamas Humane Society (2002). Personal communication.

7. Mather, J. and Fielding, W. J. (1999). A report on the ARK spay-neuter programme in New Providence with suggestions for government action. Report submitted to the Department of Agriculture, Nassau.

8. Clarkson, M. J. & Owen, L. N. (1959). The parasites of domestic animals in the Bahama islands. *Ann. Trop. Med.* 53: 341–346.

9. The Nassau Guardian (1960). The brown dog tick—a difficult pest. June 25–26, p. 10 and a follow-up article, 2–3 July, p. 10.

10. Fielding, W. J. (1999). Summary from the December/January 1998 census of veterinary clinics, New Providence. Submitted to the Department of Agriculture, The Bahamas.

11. Grieve, R. B., Glickman, L. T., Bater, A. K., Mika-Grieve, A., Thomas, C. B. and Patronek, G. J. (1986). Canine *Dirofilaria immitis* infection in a hyperenzootic area: Examination by parasitologic findings at necropsy and by two serodiagnostic methods. *American Journal of Veterinary Research* 47(2): 329–332. We know of one pack of about six roaming potcakes at Montague Beach which have died almost certainly as a result of the 2003 outbreak.

12. Higgins, D. A. (1966). Observations on the canine transmissible venereal tumour as seen in the Bahamas. *The Veterinary Record* 79(3): 67–71; Samuels, D. (2003). Personal communication.

13. Mather, Jane, Fielding, W. J. & Darling, Ingrid. (1999). Stray dogs in New Providence: An acceptable problem? *Bahamas Journal of Science* 6(2): 10–16.

14. World Health Organization (1987). *Guidelines for dog rabies control.* World Health Organization, Geneva.

15. The Tribune (2003). Pooch protection. 24 April, p. 5.

16. We know of one pack of about six roaming potcakes at Montague Beach which have died almost certainly as a result of the 2003 outbreak.

17. The Tribune (2002). Youngsters get taught a lesson in animal care. 31 July, p. 10; The Punch (2002). Spay your dog to help control stray problem. 25 February, p. 19; The Nassau Guardian (1998). The facts on stray dogs. 6 March, p. 1B

18. The Tribune (2002). Letter to the editor: Animal rights in the Bahamas, 8 May, p. 4.

19. As of 1 September 2003.

20. Some records were missing so comparative totals based on the available data were estimated, allowing for differences in monthly catch numbers.

21. The Tribune (2001). "CCU need help to tackle dog nuisance." 17 October, p. 5.

22. The Nassau Guardian (1999). Efforts increased to reduce stray dog population. 4 May, p. 4A; HSI at work in The Bahamas. www.hsus2.org/international/bahamas.html.

23. The Tribune (2003). Dogs have had their day. 15 April, pp. 1, 11; The Nassau Guardian (2003). Bain Town residents threaten dog catchers. 17 April, pp. A1, 4A.

24. For example: The Tribune (2002). Police dogs unleashed at show. 8 March, p. 9.

25. Hall, June (2002). Personal communication.

26. Mather, J. and Fielding. W. J. (1999). Op. cit.

27. Roberts, M. (2000). Personal communication. Abaco Animals Require Kindness.

28. For example: The Tribune (1998). Hope in a bus: One woman tackles Nassau's stray dog problem with kindness. 13 June, p. 12.

29. The Tribune (2002). Call to be AWARE of animal welfare. 8 February, p. 8.

30. Rotary Club Nassau Sunrise Special Supplement (2002). Who let the dogs out? March, p. 14. Published by The Tribune.

Chapter 5: What Is a "Pet"?

1. The Tribune (1924). Letter to the editor: Dumb friends of human beings? 3 May, p. 4.

2. In this section we are not interested in discussing definitions of "pet" other than in the Bahamian context. Many dictionaries and laws have defined "pet." E.g.: of a legal definition: European convention for the protection of pet animals (ETS no. 125). http://coventions.coe.int/Treaty/en/Reports/Html/125/htm.

3. These data collected were collected by Cristin Carole and used with permission.

4. We have often been told that "my" sibling has a pet or the pet is not "mine."

5. Beetz, A. (2002). Love, violence and sexuality in relationships between humans and animals. PhD thesis. Friedrich Alexander Universität Erlangen, Nürnberg.

6. The Department of Agriculture limits the types of animals which can be imported to ensure that exotic species are neither a public health hazard or potentially invasive.

7. Beetz, A. (2002). Op. cit.

8. These figures refer only to respondents from The College of The Bahamas who were included in the attachment study.

9. Beetz, A. (2002). Op. cit.

10. For example: The Tribune (1994). Two guard dogs killed at auto dealers. 2 August, pp. 1, 12.

11. The distinction between pet "owner" and "guardian" has been considered elsewhere. The Animal Policy Report (1999). Pet guardian or owner? 13(4) 3. http://www.tufts.edu/vet/cfa/13(4)nws.pdf

12. Armstrong, M. C., Tomasello, S. and Hunter, C. (2001). From pets to companion animals. In: *The state of the animals 2001*. (Eds.: Salem, D. J. and Rowan, A. N.). Humane Society Press, Washington, 71–85.

13. Beetz, A. (2002). Op. cit.

14. Beck, A. and Katcher, A. (1996). *Between pets and people: The importance of animal companionship*. Purdue University Press, West Lafayette.

15. Irwin, P. (2001). Overview: The state of animals in 2001. In: *The state of the animals 2001*. (eds. Salem, D. J. and Rowan, A. N.). Humane Society Press, Washington, 1–19.

16. See Chapter 6, on pet attachment.

17. From our resident perception study.

18. Beetz, A. (2002). Op. cit.

19. See our section on neutering.

20. Women are the head of household in 36.4% of households. Department of Statistics (2002). *Report of the 2000 census of population & housing*. Ministry of Economic Development, Nassau.

Chapter 6: Pet Attachment

1. The Tribune (2002). Letter to the editor: Animal rights in the Bahamas. 8 May, p. 4.

2. Templer, D. I., Salter, C. A., Dickey, S., Baldwin, R. and Veleber, D. M. (1981). The construction of a pet attitude scale. *The Psychological Record*. 31: 343–348. The changes made were intended to localize responses in the form. The form was made available by A. Beck and is used with permission.

3. Those who were "unsure" were omitted.

4. See the section on owned dogs.

5. These types of comments were made when we were inviting people to participate in our perception studies.

6. Albert, A. and Bulcroft, K. (1987). Pets and urban life. *Anthrozoös* 1: 9–25.

7. For example: Lookabaugh Triebenbacher, S. (1995). The relationship between attachment to companion animals and self-concept: A development perspective. 7 International Conference on Human-Animal Interactions, Animals, Health and Quality of Life, September 6–9, Geneva.

8. This is illustrated by there being only two nursing homes in New Providence listed in the telephone directory.

9. From our neutering study. The 2000 census found that the percentage of households of size one and two was 39%, while 23% such households (p<0.001) were found in the study.

10. Ministry of Economic Development (1997). *Report of the 1990 census of population and housing. Volume I Demographic and social characteristics.* Ministry of Economic Development, Nassau.

11. Department of Statistics (2002). *Report of the 2000 census of population & housing.* Ministry of Economic Development, Nassau.

12. This score allows for reversed marking of some questions, see Appendix 1.

13. Staats, S., Miller, D., Carnot, M. J., Rada, K. and Turnes, J. (1996). The Miller-Rada commitment to pets scale. *Anthrozoös* 9(2/3): 88–94.

14. Johnson, T. J., Garrity, T. F. and Stallones, L. (1992). Psychometric evaluation of the Lexington attachment to pets scale (LAPS). *Anthrozoös* 5(3): 160–175.

15. This may be explained by the fact that others have found that owners from "black" races are more attached to pets than those from "white" races. Johnson, T.P., Garrity, T. F. and Stallones, L. (1992). Op. cit.

16. Johnson, T.P., Garrity, T. F. and Stallones, L. (1992). Op. cit.

17. From our neuter study.

18. Moss, P. A. (2002). Family life. Archdiocese of Nassau 2002 Archdiocesan Assembly, 17–22 February, 2002. Archdiocesan Communications Department, Nassau. Pp. 5, 19, 20, 23.

19. The Punch (2002). A woman with two dogs and a Kemp Road gallery. 12 December, p. 28.

20. Drews, C. (2002). Attitudes, knowledge and wild animals as pets in Costa Rica. *Anthrozoös* 15 (2): 119–138.

21. Drews, C. (2002). *Op. cit.*

22. The Tribune (1998). Dog alerts family to fire, dies before they can save it. Wooden home destroyed. 7 May, pp. 1, 11.

23. The Nassau Guardian (2002). A memorial service will be held for Taco Strachan…30 August, p. 2A.

24. The Tribune (2003). Letter to the editor. 27 May, p. 4.

Chapter 7: Responsibilities of Owners Towards Pets

1. The Nassau Guardian (2001). Editorial: The stray dogs problem. 11 May, p. 8A.

2. For example, The Nassau Guardian (1993). Veterinary Assoc. points out importance of responsible animal ownership. 21 May, p. 4.

3. The Nassau Guardian (1993). Op. cit.

4. Government of The Bahamas (1987). (ed. Bryce, G.) *Statute law of the Bahamas 1799–1987*. A. Wheaton & Co. Ltd., Exeter, UK. Chapter 77.

5. Op. cit., p. 1077.

6. The Tribune (2002). Minister: we're tackling dog issue but public must help. 19 September, p. 6.

7. For comparison, information as to what is regarded as responsible dog ownership in American can be found at "Caring for Your Dog: The Top Ten Essentials" on the website of the Humane Society of the United States (2002). http://www.hsus.org/ace/11868.

8. The focus groups were conducted by Cristin Carole, Joan Vanderpool and Denise Samuels.

9. The "names" of the two interviewees are fictitious.

10. This was probably only being done due to advice given to the family by JM on a previous visit.

11. This shows that dogs will eat more than just meat and starch when garbage bins are turned over.

12. There may be the unconscious realisation that dogs such as Chihuahuas are too small to be guard dogs, and larger (guard) dogs are most effective when outside the house, to be seen and heard by strangers.

13. This conflict of views is consistent with our perception studies, where non-pet owners were more worried about catching diseases from dogs than pet owners. This is of course consistent inasmuch one would be unwilling to share the same space with a perceived health hazard.

14. Feeding table scraps is not confined to any one social group, and some people boast of feeding the "very best" leftovers to their dogs. *What's on Abaco* (1999), July, pp. 9, 21.

15. In the chapter on cruelty it will be seen that many people consider it to cruel confine their dogs.

16. See results from our surveys below.

17. These are both introduced species. The Eurasian collared dove arrived in 1975. Bainton, A. (2002). Personal communication.

18. Douglas, K. (2000). Mind of a dog. *New Scientist* 2228: 22–27.

19. Budd, T. (1999). Burglary of domestic dwellings. Findings from the British Crime Survey. The Home Office Statistical Bulletin 4/99. www.homweoffice.gov.uk/rds/pubsintro/.htm.

20. Hakim, S., Buck, A (1991). Residential security: The Hakim-Buck study on suburban alarm effectiveness. Philadelphia: Department of Economics. Temple University. www.usdoj.gov/cops/pdf/cp_resources/guidebooks/e07011182.pdf. Also see our chapter on dogs and household security.

21. The Tribune (2002). Husband and wife in home rape terror. 4 November, pp. 1, 11.

22. Also notice that he does not refer to his mongrel as a potcake. This is probably because it has many traits of the two breeds.

23. See our perception study.

24. The classic example of this is our treatment of the environment; for example, the sum of many peoples' often unnecessary or selfish use of cars has been a major contribution to global warming and climate change, from which we shall all suffer.

25. Lack of knowledge by owners on dog licensing was observed when M.I. and W.F. were photographing dogs for this publication.

26. While taking photographs of two (unlicensed) pit bull dogs on the beach, WF carelessly parked his car. A passing police car was quick to draw the poor parking to WF's attention, but the officers did not check that the dogs were licensed.

27. World Health Organization (1984). The dog population in urban and rural areas. In K. Bogel (ed.) *Guidelines for dog rabies control.* 2.1–2.38, Geneva, Switzerland.

28. Miss F. only allows the smallest of her dogs into the house. Perhaps if people bought smaller dogs, they would be more inclined to allow them inside the house than larger dogs. In some ways, a small dog always would be perceived to be a pup.

29. For example, The Tribune (2000). Packs of wild dogs pose major problem. 20 November, p. 3.

30. Veenkamp, B. (2002).Winning the dog wars. *Times of the islands. The international magazine of the Turks & Caicos.* Spring, 27–31.

31. Veenkamp, B. (2002). Op. cit.

32. See readings in Lockwood, R. and Ascione, F. R. (eds.) (1998). *Cruelty to animals and interpersonal violence.* Purdue University Press, West Lafayette.

33. Those over 35 years of age.

34. Beck, A. and Katcher, A. (1996). *Between pets and people.* Purdue University Press, West Lafayette.

Chapter 8: Roaming Dogs

Some of the material in this chapter is reused with permission from Fielding, W. J. and Mather, J. (2000). *Journal of Applied Animal Welfare Science* 3(4): 305–319.

1. The Tribune (1924). Letter to the editor: Dumb friends of human beings? 3 May, p. 4.

2. Government of the Bahamas (1988). The statute law of The Bahamas. Wheaton & Co. Ltd., Exeter. Chapter 342, p. 5209.

3. From a veterinarian, The Nassau Guardian (1998). The facts on stray dogs. 6 March, p. 1; from an activist, The Tribune (2000). Letter to the editor: Take time to think of our animal friends. 22 December, p. 4; from the government viewpoint, The Guardian (1998). Stricter legislation planned to address stray dog problem. 17 March, pp. 1A, 4A.

4. Based on our research and the number of households at the time, we feel that 45,000 was a fair estimate of owned dogs. We link the owned and unowned dog populations to the number of households. As the number of households increase, all other things being equal, we would expect the number of roaming dogs to also increase. For issues related to dog ownership in The Bahamas, see Chapter 10. JM was a member of this committee. The inaccurate press report in The Nassau Guardian (1998). Unit struggles to control island's 45,000 stray dogs. 23 May, p. 7A.

5. The Tribune (2000). Packs of wild dogs pose major problem. 20 November, p. 3.

6. The Tribune (2001). Campaigner seeks end to potcake problem. 10 May, p. 2.

7. For example: Male owners are less likely to neuter their dogs in Australia. See Chapter 12.

8. Since the mid-seventies, the word "cur" seems to have been replaced by "potcake" in press reports. See Chapter 3.

9. For example: The Tribune (2000). Packs of wild dogs pose major problem. 20 November, p. 3.

10. Our observations of dogs in the Kemp Road area indicate that 4% of the roaming dogs had collars.

11. The importance of abandonment in maintaining the roaming dog is discussed in further detail later.

12. The Guardian (1991). Vet: owners should restrain dogs. 15 February, p. 4A.

13. The Tribune (2000). Potcakes growing more confident. 9 November, p. 1.

14. See the discussion concerning "breed" dogs in the next chapter.

15. Fielding, W. J. (2000). A study on cats and dogs in Marsh Harbour and Nassau. *Bahamas Journal of Science* 7(2): 27–34.

16. Just because no pedigree-type dog was seen, we cannot say that all roaming dogs are potcakes, as we may have missed some non-potcakes. Casley, D., and Kumar, K. (1988). *The collection, analysis, and use of monitoring and evaluation data.* Johns Hopkins University Press.

17. The Tribune (2000). Valiant friend looking for health restoration. 15 July, p. 9. Such observations are to be expected in light of the breeds of dogs imported in Table 10.1.

18. Although the Bahamas Kennel Club does not recognise the pit bull as a breed, people typically consider pit bulls as a breed. "Calvin [a potcake] with possible pitbull relations, went on to become both a vigilant watchdog . . ." Kerr, J. (undated). Potcakes. The great dogs of the Abaco islands. Abaco Life. http://go-abacos.com/news/ablife/news_contd2.htlm.

19. The Punch (2002). Letter to the editor. 19 August, p. 38. (Emphasis original.)

20. We were unable to find out which animals had been surrendered or caught.

21. Beck, A. M. (1973). The ecology of stray dogs. A study of free-ranging urban animals. Purdue University Press, reprinted 2002.

22. Beck, A. M. (2000). Personal communication.

23. Boitani, L., Francisci, F., Ciucci, P. and Andreoli, G. (1995). Population biology and ecology of feral dogs in central Italy. In: *The domestic dog: its evolution, behaviour and interactions with people.* (ed. Serpell, J.). Cambridge University Press, 217–244.

24. For example: The Nassau Guardian (2001). Animal rights activists want GBI stray animals neutered. 10 May, p. 12A.

25. A group of (legally) owned, roaming dogs were monitored between October 2001 and August 2003. As the dogs were kept on private property we could only view them at a distance or when they were roaming. The observations confirm the inability of such dogs to increase their numbers, even with almost daily human interaction. These animals were brought to a building site to protect construction materials. A worker fed the

animals regularly and visited the site at weekends. Prior to the start of this observation, the female had had puppies at least twice before, but only two puppies appeared to have survived in about 2.5 years, prior to October 2001 (we assume that no animals were removed from the site). Then she had had a litter of unknown size in August 2001. A car killed (at least) one of the animals and two were poisoned (September 2001) (reported by a neighbour). By October 2001 two adults and only two puppies could be seen, one puppy from the last litter and one puppy from an earlier litter. Two litters were produced, in early and late 2002. A close encounter showed that one of the young dogs was blind in one eye (December 2001). Only one puppy from the latter litter was heard by late-December (probably born in late November); one other surviving puppy had been found and taken to the Bahamas Humane Society by a neighbour. By October 2002, only one of the original dogs was seen. The change in group size is given in Figure 33F.

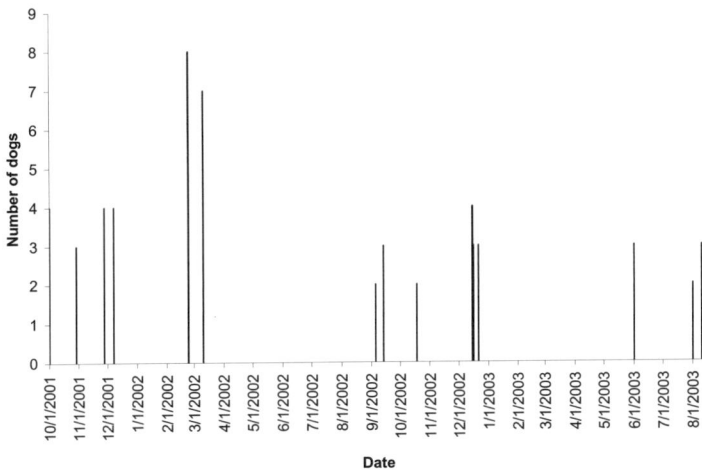

Figure 33F: Group size of owned, roaming dogs on a building site, West Bay Street between 2001 and 2003.

26. It also questions the fecundity associated with potcakes.

27. Grieve, R. B., Glickman, L. T., Bater, A. K., Mika-Grieve, A., Thomas, C. B. and Patronek, G. J. (1986). Canine Dirofilaria immitis infection in a hyperenzootic area: Examination by parasitologic findings at necropsy and by two serodiagnostic methods. American Journal of Veterinary Research 47(2): 329–332.

28. Provox (2001). The publicity voice of the Rotary Club of Providenciales 38(3) p. 1.

29. Mather, J. and Fielding W. J. (1999). Op. cit.

30. See our "Balance Sheet," Table 25.

31. About 1% more than at the start of the year, as this is the estimated growth in household numbers by the Department of Statistics.

32. See Figure 10.2.

33. For example: The Tribune (2001). Op. cit.

34. The Freeport News (2000). Increase of stray animals in GB. 1 March, pp. 8, 9.

35. The Tribune (2001). New bid to keep dogs at bay. Independence Supplement, p. 3.

36. Beck, A. M. (1973). Op. cit.

37. This is an expanded version of a figure first published in the *Bahamas Journal of Science*. Fielding, W. J. (2003). Letter to the editor: Perceptions of the size of the roaming dog population. *Bahamas Journal of Science* 10(2): 43.

38. Beck (1973) has shown how increased human activity reduces the number of dogs seen on the streets. In Nassau, human activity is markedly different during and outside school terms, both in terms of fewer pedestrians and cars. Hence the need to take comparable observations during term time.

39. This is higher than the percentage of tourists who felt that The Bahamas had a "stray dog problem." See Chapter 9.

40. Saunders, T., and Storr, D. (2002). Roaming dogs. Unpublished research project for Course 421, Man and the Environment, The College of The Bahamas. A possible explanation for the differences in these responses could be that Bain Town is socio-economically poorer, dwelling are less likely to be enclosed, and the area probably has a higher crime rate than Yamacraw.

41. Fielding, W. J. (1999). Perceptions of owned and unowned animals: A case study from New Providence. *Bahamas Journal of Science* 6(2): 17–22.

42. Saunders, T., and Storr, D. (2002). Op. cit.

43. Fielding, W. J. (2000). Enquiries into dog ownership in Abaco with specific reference to AARF/SNIP. Submitted to the Humane Society of the United States (HSUS), Washington, DC.

44. See Chapter 9.

45. Some actions of residents towards roaming dogs are mentioned in Chapter 14.

46. Saunders, T., and Storr, D. (2002). Op. cit.

47. The Nassau Guardian (2003). Bain Town residents threaten dog catchers. 17 April, pp. A1, 4A.

48. Matter, H. C. and Daniels, T. J. (2000). Dog ecology and population biology. In: Macpherson, C. N. L., Meslin, F. X. and Wandeler, A. I. (eds.) *Dogs, zoonoses, and public health*. CABI, UK, 17–62.

49. The potcake's bark has been compared to that of the noise of a hurricane; see This week on: fredmitchelluncensored.com, 11 November, 2001. In Bain Town 71% (of 35 respondents) complained about garbage being split, as did 80% in Yamacraw. Saunders, T., and Storr, D. (2002). Op. cit. From time to time, the Department of Agriculture receives complaints of roaming dogs attacking livestock. Such reports have apparently decreased in recent years, as less livestock farming is carried out in New Providence. On other islands with more farming, dog attacks are reported occasionally.

50. Other complaints reported by those who actually suffered nuisances were: faeces, 33%; nuisance due to dogs being a health hazard, 11%; mating, 9%; trespassing on property,

8%; damage to property, 7.4%. Twenty-two percent reported "other" nuisances such as the dogs being a danger on the roads, roaming in packs and attacking people.

51. Government of the Bahamas (1988). *The statute law of The Bahamas* Vol. II. Wheaton & Co. Ltd., Exeter; Government of the Bahamas (1988). *The statute law of The Bahamas* Vol. V. Wheaton & Co. Ltd., Exeter; Government of the Bahamas (1989). *The subsidiary legislation of The Bahamas* Vol. IV. BPCC Wheaton Ltd., Exeter.

52. Allen, D. (2000). Personal communication. Public Health Inspectorate, Nassau.

53. Stanley International (1996). *Bahamas solid waste and hazardous material management project, Pre-investment report. Mid-term report.* Stanley International, Edmonton, Alberta.

54. This is the number we have estimated for the free-roaming population in New Providence, based on the perception study.

55. Fielding, W. J. (1999). Perceptions of owned and unowned animals: A case study from New Providence. *Bahamas Journal of Science* 6(2): 17–22.

56. We disagree with media reports that give the impression that large numbers of roaming dogs "shuffle along the street, no more than bare skin stretched over bone." The Punch (2003). Minister Pratt's prison plan for inmates right on target. 8 May, page. 16.

57. McKenzie, T. (2002). Rodent problem can only be curbed through "education." The Nassau Guardian. http://nas.bits.baseview.com/nas_templates/print/27649904302439.nas.

58. The Tribune (1998). 20,000 rats take over Bay Street straw market. 22 May, p. 1.

59. Rolle, L. (2000). Personal communication, Department of Housing, Nassau.

60. McPherson, C. (2000). Personal communication. St. George's University, Granada.

61. Data on hotels, restaurants, and supermarkets from Stanley International (1996). Op. cit. Food containers found in roadside garbage and elsewhere can become breeding places for mosquitoes and other larvae, thus contributing to heart worm, dengue fever, etc.

62. The Tribune (2000). On-going plan to keep out rabies. 9 May, p. 5.

63. For example: The Nassau Guardian (1998). The facts on stray dogs. 6 March, p. 1B.

64. From our resident perception study in New Providence.

65. Potter, R. (1993). The neglect of Caribbean vernacular architecture. *Bahamas Journal of Science.* 1(1) 46–51.

66. Sawyer, A. (2002). Bahamian perceptions, attitudes and beliefs on animal cruelty. Student study for SOS 200, Independent research, School of Social Sciences, The College of The Bahamas. (Note: some of the data presented by us does not appear in her report.) Data used with permission.

67. These dogs are probably a rare an example of community-owned dogs that receive veterinary care in addition to merely being fed.

68. Ownership, even within a household, is often personalised. Household members can live in a dog-owning household but do not necessarily consider themselves as a dog owner, or as having responsibilities towards the animal.

69. The Nassau Guardian (1999). Public opinion. 27 April. Probably p. 8A. (Department of Archives microfilm incomplete.)

70. Matter, H. C. and Daniels, T. J. (2000). Dog ecology and population biology. In: *Dogs, zoonoses and public health* (ed. Macpherson, C. N. L., Meslin, F. X., and Wandeler, A. I.). CABI Publishing, 17–62.

71. Matter, H. C. and Daniels, T. J. (2000). Op. cit.

Chapter 9: Tourists and Roaming Dogs

This chapter draws upon Plumridge, S. and Fielding, W. J. (unpublished) Tourists' reactions to roaming dogs in New Providence, The Bahamas.

1. The Tribune (2003). Tourist in dog attack horror. 29 January, pp. 1 and 11.

2. The Nassau Guardian (1969). Letter to the editor. 29 January, p. 4; The Nassau Guardian (1960). Letter to the editor. 11 January, p. 6.

3. The Nassau Guardian (1970). Letter to the editor. 10 April, p. 4.

4. The Nassau Guardian (2003). Our country's tourism: where do we go from here? 18 February. http://archive.nassauguardian.net/archive_detail.php?archiveFile=./pubfiles/&archive_pubname=. Accessed 28 April 2003.

5. The Tribune (2003) Tourist dog attack 'could have been avoided'. 30 January, pp. 1, 11.

6. The Nassau Guardian (2003). Stray dogs threaten tourism, Wilchcombe says. Pp. 1A, 11A.

7. The Tribune (2002). Let's grow out of this backward potcake culture. 18 February, p. 5.

8. The Bahama Journal (2003). Potcake dogs finding love in foreign homes. 12 August. http://www.jonescommunicationsltd.com/journal/index.php?url_channel_id=0&url_subchannel_id_&url_publish_channel_id=159&well_id=2

9. The Tribune (1999). Stray dogs: A complicated problem. 25 February, p. 10.

10. The Nassau Guardian (2003). Checking the Bahamian visitor profile. Pp. B1, B2.

11. Anon (1999). Effect of stray dogs on tourists: Summary of pilot study in New Providence, March. Presented to the Department of Agriculture's Stray dog committee.

12. Comments from tourists in this study.

13. BBC News (2001). Greek dogs find Olympic hero. 31 March. http://news.bbc.co.uk/2/hi/europe/1251619.stm

14. Bahamas Environment, Science and Technology (BEST) Commission (1998). Draft national report. To the Conference of the Parties to the Convention on Biological Diversity. BEST Commission, Nassau.

15. We know of tourists who have been bitten by dogs and were almost terrified of catching rabies, although Nassau remains rabies-free.

16. Letters to the Editor: Bahamarama NSNBCNews (undated). http://www.msnbc.com/news/849177.asp?cp1=1#BODY. Accessed 5 February 2003.

17. People for the Ethical treatment of Animals (Undated). Action Alerts. The Bahamas: No Paradise for dogs. http://www.peta.org/alert/automation/AlertItem.asp?id=588.

18. The Nassau Guardian (2003). Checking the Bahamian visitor profile. Pp. B1, B2.

19. Harper, J (2001). Road Worriers. Insight on the News, 10/1/2001, 17 Issue 37, p. 33.

20. Plumridge, S. and Fielding, W. J. (unpublished). Tourists' reactions to roaming dogs in New Providence, The Bahamas.

21. Ralston Purina (2000). The state of the American pet: A study among pet owners. http://www.purina.com/images/articles/pdf/TheStateofThe.pdf.

22. Saunders, T., and Storr, D. (unpublished). Roaming dogs. Edu 421 Man & the environment. The College of The Bahamas, student project, 2002.

23. Beck, A. (1973). The ecology of stray dogs. A study of free-ranging urban animals. Reprinted 2002. Purdue University Press.

24. It should also be recalled that some Bahamians do not like to see dogs being caught by animal control officers.

25. The Tribune (2003). 'Many, many groups' tacking stray dogs problem. 28 January, p. 5.

26. Anon (undated). The islands of The Bahamas. Exit study report. Stopover customer evaluation. Main findings. Full year 2001. Bahamas Ministry of Tourism.

27. The Tribune (2003). Child injured in pig attack terror. 16 July, pp. 1, 11.

Chapter 10: Owned Dogs

Some of the material in this chaptered is reused with permission and appeared in Fielding, W. J. and Mather, J. (2000), *Journal of Applied Animal Welfare Science* 3(4): 305–319; Fielding, W. J. and Mather, J. (2001), Dog Ownership in the West Indies: A case study from The Bahamas, *Anthrozoös* 14(2): 72–80; and Fielding, W. J. and Mather (2002), *College of The Bahamas Research Journal* 11: 41–56.

1. The Tribune (2001). Editorial: Stray dog problem—solution needed. 26 September, p. 4.

2. Dog License. Chapter 342, p. 5207.

3. Op. cit.

4. Insufficient dog license tags are distributed, so not all dogs can be licensed. Fielding, W. J. (2000). Some observations on licensed dogs. Submitted to the Department of Agriculture, The Bahamas.

5. Anon (undated). Legislation dog owners should know. Department of Agriculture information sheet.

6. Anon (undated). Legislation dog owners should know. Op. cit.

7. If this were the correct figure, over twice as many license tags would have to be distributed than were made available in 1999. Fielding, W. J. (2000). Op. cit. Some owners think that their dog only needs to be licensed once, rather than each year.

8. In Kemp Road. Fielding, W. J. (2003). Unpublished data.

9. It should be noted that not all these dogs would be permanent members of the Bahamian dog population, as foreign dogs which enter the Bahamas Kennel Club shows are also registered. Hall, R. (2002). Personal communication.

10. Hall, R. (2002). Personal communication.

11. See Chapter 11.

12. Such dogs are omitted from the breeds listed in Table 10.1.

13. However, it should be noted that these animals may not be "pure" or registered.

14. Fielding, W. J. (2002). Unpublished data.

15. We note that in 1988, female pit bulls cost $350 and males $300. This suggests that there is still considerable demand for them despite the large number of advertisements. The Tribune (1988). Pets for sale. 2 November, p. 10.

16. Fielding, W. J. (unpublished data). Advertisements in the two daily newspapers were monitored between November 2002 and early March 2003.

17. Many of these aspects are similar in Marsh Harbour, Abaco. Fielding, W. J. (2000). A study of cats and dogs in Marsh Harbour and Nassau. *Bahamas Journal of Science* 7(2): 27–34.

18. Humane Society International (2001). Dogs on Abaco island, The Bahamas. A case study. Humane Society International, Washington, DC.

19. If dogs were evenly distributed throughout the population, the line would be a straight line at 45 degrees, from the bottom left corner to the top right corner of the graph. The more the curve deviates from this line, the greater the disparity in the ownership.

20. From our neuter study.

21. World Health Organisation (1988). *Report of WHO consultation on dog ecology studies related to rabies control. Geneva, 22–25 February 1988.* Geneva, World Health Organization.

22. Saunders, T., and Storr, D. (2002). Roaming dogs. Unpublished research project for Course 421, Man and the Environment, The College of The Bahamas.

23. Patronek, G. J., Beck, A. M. and Glickman, L. T. (1997). Dynamics of dog and cat populations in a community. *JAVMA* 210(5): 637–642.

24. Drews, C. (2001). Wild animals and other pets kept in Costa Rican households: incidence, species and numbers. *Society & Animals* 9(2): 107–126.

25. World Health Organisation (1988). *Report of WHO consultation on dog ecology studies related to rabies control. Geneva, 22–25 February 1988.* Geneva, World Health Organization.

26. Saunders, T., and Storr, D. (2002). Op. cit.

27. The Nassau Guardian. (2002). Wise forethought best weapon against crime. Httl://nas.baseview.com/nas_templates/search/2780004794082.nas (2 October 2002).

28. For example, www.biminilove.org/potcake.html.

29. The Tribune (1998). Dog alerts family to fire, dies before they can save it. Wooden home destroyed. 7 May, pp. 1, 11.

30. From our neuter study; see Chapter 12.

31. From our neuter study; see Chapter 12.

32. Fielding, W. J., (2000). Enquiries into dog ownership in Abaco with specific reference to AARF/SNIP. Submitted to the Humane Society of the United States (HSUS), Washington, DC.

33. Humane Society International (2001). *Dogs on Abaco island, The Bahamas. A case study.* Humane Society International, Washington, DC.

34. Sawyer, A. (2002). Bahamian perceptions, attitudes and beliefs on animal cruelty. Student study for SOS 200, Independent research, School of Social Sciences, The College of The Bahamas.

35. American Kennel Club. http://www.akc.org/breeds/index.cfm.

36. Turnquest, S. (2001). Personal communication. Bahamas Humane Society, Nassau.

37. Although the pit bull is not recognised as a "breed" as such by the American Kennel Club (http://www.akc.org/breeds/index.cfm), in New Providence it would be considered as a "breed" animal by most dog owners.

38. The Tribune (2000). Close encounters with . . . Dr. Peter Bizzell. 28 August, p. 1C.

39. Fielding, W. J., (2000). Enquiries into dog ownership in Abaco with specific reference to AARF/SNIP. Submitted to the Humane Society of the United States (HSUS), Washington, DC.

40. We recognise that age and quality of life are not synonymous and that animals can live miserable lives for a long time.

41. In Abaco only.

42. On Barbados, see World Health Organisation (1979). Animal and human health. Report for the Government of Barbados, BAR/78/002/A/01/4. United Nations Development Programme; on Tunisia, see World Health Organisation (1988). *Report of WHO consultation on dog ecology studies related to rabies control. Geneva, 22–25 February 1988.* Geneva, World Health Organization.

43. Patronek, G. J., Beck, A. M. and Glickman, L. T. (1997). Op. cit.

44. The Economist (2002). It's a dog's life. December 21, 2002–January 3, 2003, 61–63.

45. Mather, J., Fielding, W. J. and Darling, I. (1999). Op. cit.

46. The Nassau Guardian (2001). Five charged with having sex with 13-year-old girl, 27 June http://www.bamainfo.com/news_display.php?prid=551&scr=nassau.

47. The breeding of pit bulls can be expected to be popular, as the government does not issue import permits for them.

48. From our study on neutering.

49. Our observations from Abaco.

50. An average of 42 dogs a week is collected by Solid Waste, the unit responsible for collecting dead animals. Most of these dogs are killed by cars. Data especially collected for us. Hepburn, L. (2000). Department of Environmental Health, Nassau.

51. Most of the observations in this section are from Abaco.

52. This figure compares with results from a study on youth health that found that at least 36% had never been or could not remember going to a doctor, and at least 36% had never been or could not remember going to a dentist. Health Information Unit (2001). Bahamas Youth health survey, Ministry of Health, Nassau. Unpublished.

53. Observations from New Providence.

54. Fielding. W. J. (2000). Enquiries into dog ownership in Abaco with specific reference to AARF/SNIP. Submitted to the Humane Society of the United States (HSUS), Washington, DC.

55. From our 1998 perception study in New Providence.

56. Fielding, W. J. (2000). Enquiries into dog ownership in Abaco with specific reference to AARF/SNIP. Submitted to the Humane Society of the United States (HSUS), Washington, DC.

57. Serpell, J., and Jagoe, J. A. (1995). Early experience and the development of behaviour. In: *The domestic dog: Its evolution, behaviour and interactions with people* (ed. Serpell, J.). Cambridge University Press, 79–102.

58. For example: What is a potcake? www.biminilove.org/potcake.html. Accessed 5 June 2003.

59. Fielding, W. J. (2000). A study of roaming dogs in Abaco, The Bahamas. Submitted to the Humane Society of the United States, Washington, DC.

60. Fielding, W. J. (2000). A study of roaming dogs in Abaco, The Bahamas. Submitted to the Humane Society of the United States, Washington, DC.

61. Manning, A. M., and Rowan, A. N. (1992). Companion animal demographics and sterilization status: Results from a survey in four Massachusetts towns. *Anthrozoös* 5:192–201.

62. Department of Statistics (2002). Report of the 2000 census of population and housing. Ministry of Economic Development, Nassau.

63. The Tribune (2002). Drinking water fears over Haitian shanty settlement. 29 October, pp. 1, 11.

64. This is not an unusual reaction. Rowan, A. (1999). Personal communication.

65. Owners consider abandoning the dog in this way as "giving it a chance"; if they surrender the animal they "know" it will die.

66. It should be remembered that the Animal Control Unit is the only organisation charged with seizing unwanted animals and that it passes adoptable animals to the Bahamas Humane Society. The Bahamas Humane Society does not collect dogs. The comment indicates the automatic link that people make between the Animal Control Unit and the death of an animal.

67. Fielding, W. J. (2000). A study of roaming dogs in Abaco, The Bahamas. Submitted to the Humane Society of the United States, Washington, DC.

68. See the interpretation of Miss F. in the case study in Chapter 7.

69. We often hear people say, "He cannot really get out" or "She just goes down the road and back again" or "She just gets out for a moment."

70. Anon (undated). Legislation dog owners should know. Department of Agriculture information sheet. It should also be noted that in 1965, the fine was £25 or about $475 at today's value. Government of Bahamas (1965). *Bahamas Acts passed in the 1965.* Nassau Guardian.

71. The Punch (2002). Letter to the editor: Owners need to keep fierce dogs locked in yards! 19 August, p. 38. The letter lists Akitas, Great Danes, as well as pit bulls as roaming in Winton Heights, in the east of the island.

72. World Health Organisation (1988). *Report of WHO consultation on dog ecology studies related to rabies control. Geneva, 22–25 February 1988.* Geneva, World Health Organization.

73. From Saunders, T., and Storr, D. (2002). Op. cit.

74. There was no significant difference in the responses in Bain Town (69%) and Yamacraw (74%), p>0.05.

75. The same percentage was reported in both Bain Town and Yamacraw.

76. In South Africa, abandonment was the second most common cause of animal abuse, showing that The Bahamas is not singular in abandoning animals. Vermeulen, H., and Odendaal, J. S. J. (1993). Op. cit.

77. Rolle points to an all-too-common procedure of disposing of unwanted pets—rather than surrendering the dogs to local authorities, some owners simply drive to bushy, less inhabited spots and dump their once-treasured pet, like an old rusting refrigerator. She describes one man's method, possibly an all-too-common one, of getting rid of an un-wanted pet:

> He said he drove out and dropped the dog off where the dog couldn't find home. So I said "why did you do that? That's a very unkind thing to do to an animal!" He said he dropped it in an area where there's a lot of people, so the dog would be fed. But there's no guarantee that the dog would be fed if you drop it in an area where there are a lot of people, because there might be a lot of people in the area just like you, that don't want to be bothered with a dog. The Nassau Guardian (2001). Animal Care. 18 September. http://www.bahamainfo.com/news_display.php?prid=1409&src =nassau.

78. See Miss F.'s comments in Chapter 7.

79. "Advertisement: $500 reward . . . for return of female brindle pitbull puppy . . . last seen . . . around the intersection of Fifth Terrace, Centreville and East Avenue . . ." The Trib-une (2002), 27 September. P. 19.

80. About 1,250 import permits are issued annually; the actual number of dogs brought in on an import permit may be less than the number permitted, which could be as many as six. However, most of these permits are for tourists, and some temporary residents make multiple entries and exits with the same dogs, which further complicates the pic-ture. About 15% of all permits seem to be for residents and the mean number of dogs requested per permit is 1.54 (se: 0.132). Fielding, W. J. (2002). Unpublished data.

81. Beck, A. M. (1973). Op. cit.

Chapter 11: The Role of Dogs in Household Security

Some of the material in this chapter appeared in Fielding, W. J. & Plumridge, S. J. (2004). Preliminary observations of the role of dogs in household security in New Providence, The Bahamas. *Anthrozoös* 17 (2): 167–178. Used with permission.

1. The Nassau Guardian (2003). Imported personal protection . . . Classified advertisement. 29 April, p. 13B.

2. Interestingly, not all respondents knew what breeds of dog they had in the household, or their sex or breeding status.

3. See Chapter 12 for further discussion on neutering.

4. The Punch (2002). Letter to the editor. 19 August, p. 38.

5. The Punch (2003). Security alert as thugs kill judge's four guard dogs. 28 July, p. 1.

6. The Tribune (2003). Letter to the editor. 27 May, p. 4.

7. Nova, T. (undated). Choosing the best dog for protection. A comprehensive guide for the homeowner or apartment dweller. http://animalcareuse.org/article_bestdog.htlm.

8. Hert, B. L. (1995). Analysing breed and gender differences in behaviour. Pp. 66–77. In: *The domestic dog: Its evolution, behaviour and interactions with people* (ed. Serpell, J.). Cambridge University Press.

9. Lockwood, R. (1995). The ethology and epidemiology of canine aggression. Pp. 132–138. In: *The domestic dog: Its evolution, behaviour and interactions with people* (ed. Serpell, J.). Cambridge University Press.

10. For example, The Tribune (2000). Packs of wild dogs pose major problem. 20 November, p. 3; and The Nassau Guardian (2003). Stray dogs threaten tourism, Wilchcombe says. http://nas.bits.baseview.com/nas_templates/search/294647784040104.nas#.

11. The Punch (2003). Roaming dogs problem at critical stage, says BHS. 3 February, p. 9.

12. Beck, A. (1973). *The ecology of stray dogs. A study of free-roaming urban animals.* Reprinted 2002, Purdue University Press.

13. See Chapter 16.

14. Lockwood, R. (1995). Op. cit.

15. About 86% of attacks on homes take place during the day. (Personal communication, Royal Bahamas Police Force, 2003).

16. The Tribune (2002). Husband and wife in home rape terror. 4 November, pp. 1, 11.

17. Department of Statistics (1999). *Statistical abstract 1999.* Ministry of Economic Development, Nassau.

18. Department of Statistics (2002). *Report of the 2000 census of population and housing.* Ministry of Economic Development, Nassau.

Chapter 12: Attitudes and Actions towards Neutering

Some of the material in this chapter appeared in Fielding, W. J., Samuels, D. & Mather, J. (2002). Attitudes and actions of West Indian dog owners towards neutering their animals: A gender issue? *Anthrozoös* 15 (3): 206–226. Used with permission.

1. The Tribune (1999). Stray dogs: A complicated problem. 25 February, p. 10.

2. We are not sure what this means, as they could not have been legally bred in Germany and imported.

3. The Nassau Guardian (2003). Pets for sale. 5 June, p. B13. These animals varied in price from $200 to $600 each. It should be noted that potcakes are rarely advertised.

4. From our perception study.

5. Armstrong, M. C., Tomasello, S. & Hunter, C. (2001). From pets to companion animals. In *The state of the animals 2001.* (ed. Salem, D. J. & Rowan, A. N.). Humane Society Press, Washington. 71–85.

6. The Tribune (2001). Campaigner seeks end to potcake problem. 10 May, p. 2.

7. Blackshaw, J. K., & Day, C. (1994). Attitudes of dog owners to neutering pets: Demographic data and effects of owner attitudes. *Australian Veterinary Journal* 71(4): 113–116; Balfe, P. (2001). Personal communication. Veterinarian, Nassau.

8. For example, some gender differences with respect to pet attachment; see Chapter 6.

9. For example, Miura, A., Bradshaw, J. W. S., and Tanida, H. (2000). Attitudes towards dogs: A study of university students in Japan and the UK. *Anthrozoös* 13: 80–88.

10. From our perception study in New Providence.

11. WF's daughter competed in the Primary Schools' Chess Tournament (June 2001). One of her male opponents refused to play her because she was a girl, and defaulted the game. The friend of a boy whom she had just beaten asked to play her in an unofficial game; after she had also beaten him, he turned to his friend and said, "Don't tell Mister So-and-so that I lost to a girl."

12. The Nassau Guardian (2001). Editorial: Double standards for girls. 27 November, p. 6A.

13. McCartney, T. (1976). *Bahamian sexuality*. Timpaul Publishing Co., Nassau, p. 35.

14. McCartney, T. (1971). *Neurosis in the sun*. Executive Printers of the Bahamas, Ltd., p. 141.

15. BBC News (2001). Greek dogs find Olympic hero. 31 March. http://news.bbc.co.uk/2/hi/europe/1251619.stm.

16. A detailed report on this study is reported by Fielding, W. J., Samuels, D. & Mather, J. (2002). Op. cit.

17. Blackshaw, J. K., & Day, C. (1994). Op. cit.

18. The odds ratio can be used in retrospective case-control type studies when selection is based on the outcome. Altman, D. (1991). *Practical statistics for medical research*. Chapman & Hall/CRC.

19. Humane Society International (2001). *Dogs on Abaco Island, The Bahamas. A case study*. Humane Society International, Washington; Ralston Purina (2000). The state of the American pet—A study among pet owners. http://www.purina.com. On Australia, see Blackshaw & Day (1994). Op. cit.

20. Humane Society International (2001). Op. cit.

21. Blackshaw & Day (1994). Op. cit.

22. Statistics from Patronek, Beck and Glickman (1997); and Ralston Purina (2000). Op. cit., respectively.

23. On Massachusetts, see Manning, A. M., and Rowan, A. N. (1992). Companion animal demographics and sterilization status: Results from a survey in four Massachusetts towns. *Anthrozoös* 5:192–201; on Brisbane, see Blackshaw & Day (1994). Op. cit.

24. Maarschalkerweerd R. J., Endenburg, N., Kirpensteijn J., & Knol, B. W. (1997). Influence of orchiectomy on canine behaviour. *The Veterinary Record*. 617–619.

25. Blackshaw & Day (1994). Op. cit.

26. The Tribune (2001). Editorial: Stray dog problem—solution needed. 26 September, p. 4.

27. From our perception study in New Providence.

28. Blackshaw & Day (1994). Op. cit.

29. Manning and Rowan (1992). Op cit.

30. On the US, see Ralston Purina (2000). Op. cit.; on Australia, see Blackshaw & Day (1994). Op. cit.

31. Data from our study on household security; see Chapter 11.

32. Ralston Purina (2000). Op. cit.

33. Richards, M., (2001). Vetinfo. A Veterinary Information Service. www.vetinfo.com/dspay.html.

34. Animal Sheltering (2001). Profiling pets and their relinquishers. March–April, pp. 9–10.

35. Based on our observations.

36. This is usually an unstated perception, as neuter programmes tend to be aimed at poorer people, who are considered to be the ones who do not have their animals neutered. While this is true, such programmes are difficult to sustain due to the need for constant fund raising.

37. The Tribune (2002). Prized pooches take top awards. 26 July, p. 12.

38. In our pet attachment study, younger students (those 21 years or younger) were less likely to agree that pets should be treated with the same respect as humans (64% of 84), compared with other students (82% of 67) (p=0.018). This might mean that younger members of society may be more willing to neuter their pets.

39. This figure is also close to the 43% of owners who let their dogs roam in Sawyer's cruelty study.

Chapter 13: Economic Aspects of Dog Ownership

1. The Nassau Guardian (1998). Letter to the editor: Stray dogs not restricted to Over The Hill. 4 June, p. 2.

2. This is distinct to acquiring a dog. Potcakes are often given away; we know of one pet shop that gives away potcakes, so making them, by definition, "valueless."

3. Department of Statistics (2002). *Report of the 2000 census of population and housing.* Ministry of Economic Development, Nassau.

4. It should be noted that valuable animals have sometimes been found abandoned, which suggests that richer households may also abandon unwanted animals.

5. We know of many owners who have acquired potcakes just by capturing roaming dogs.

6. Eisner, M. (2001). Modernisation, self-control and lethal violence. The long-term dynamics of European homicide rates in theoretical perspective. *The British Journal of Criminology* 41: 613–638.

Chapter 14: Cruelty to Dogs

1. The Tribune (1924). Recently organised Bahamas Humane Society. 10 December, p. 6.

2. The Nassau Guardian (1989). Society officers rail against animal cruelty. 16 June, pp. A1, A4.

3. The Nassau Guardian (1892). Editorial. 26 October, p. 2.

4. Government of The Bahamas (1987). (Ed. Bryce, G.) *Statute law of the Bahamas 1799–1987.* A. Wheaton & Co. Ltd., Exeter, UK. Penal code. Chapter 77. Pp. 1077, 1099.

5. Anon (undated). Legislation dog owners should know. Department of Agriculture information sheet.

6. Rowan, A. N. (1999). Cruelty and abuse to animals. In: *Child abuse, domestic violence and animal abuse* (Ascione, F. R. & Arkow, P., eds.) Purdue University Press, 328–334.

7. Hills, A. M. and Lalich, N. (1998). Judgments of cruelty towards animals: sex differences and effect of awareness of suffering. *Anthrozoös* 11(3): 142–147.

8. Sawyer, A. (2002). Bahamian perceptions, attitudes and beliefs on animal cruelty. Independent Research Semester: 042002. The College of The Bahamas. Unpublished. Note: much of the information quoted from her study comes from our analysis of her data set and was not reported in her paper.

9. The Tribune (2000). Two charged with dog baiting. 20 September, pp. 1, 11; The Tribune (1994). Letter to the editor: Don't have to be cruel to train dogs to be 'bad'. 29 June, p. 4; The Tribune (1994). Two guard dogs killed at auto dealers. 2 August, pp. 1, 12.

10. See Chapter 11.

11. The Nassau Guardian (2002). Letter to the editor: Residents censure Pitrone—and his dog. http://nas.baseview.com/nas_templates/print/276496799355260.nas.

12. The Tribune (2000). Pets in danger from poisoners. 12 May, p. 4.

13. The Tribune (2001). Our pets were deliberately poisoned, say dog owners. 29 October, p. 3; The Tribune (2001). Pitbull infiltration 'making our potcakes turn vicious'. 4 October, p. 8.

14. The Daily Telegraph (2002). Paradise lost. 12 October, pp. 9–10.

15. The Tribune (2002). Residents are barking mad over fireworks noise. 29 October, p. 6.

16. The Tribune (2002). Training the owners of 'man's best friend'. Close encounters with…June Hall. 29 April, pp. 1C, 2C.

17. Turnquest, S. (2000). Personal communication. Bahamas Humane Society.

18. Vermeulen, H. & Odendaal, J. S. J. (1993). Proposed typology for companion animal abuse. *Anthrozoös* 6(4): 248–57.

19. Sawyer, A. (2002). *Op. cit*

20. Bahamas Handbook 2001. (2000). Etienne Dupuch Jr. Publications, Nassau.

21. The Tribune (2001). "CCU need help to tackle dog nuisance." 17 October, p. 5.

22. The Nassau Guardian (2003). Bain Town residents threaten dog catchers. 17 April, p. 1.

23. The Tribune (2000). Pets in danger from poisoners. 12 May, p. 3; The Tribune (1997). Burnt animals (dogs) by acid fire. 15 July. Pp. 1, 9.

24. The son of the man who shot the dog related this story to school friends, and so could be an example of peers indicating that sort of behaviour is acceptable.

25. The Tribune (1980). Briland has rash of dog poisonings. 25 February, p. 1.

26. Saunders, T., & Storr, D. (2002). Roaming dogs. Unpublished research project for Course 421, Man and the Environment, The College of the Bahamas.

27. Sawyer, A. (2002). *Op. cit*

28. In interviews some people talk of "running" or "shooing" dogs from their yard. Such actions might be accompanied by some sort of projectile.

29. The Nassau Guardian (1989). Society officers rail against animal cruelty. 16 June, Pp. A1, A4.

30. Sawyer, A. (2002). Op. cit.

31. Table 14.1 derived from Sawyer (2002), but does not appear in her report. Op. cit.

32. Sawyer, A. (2002). Op. cit.

33. The story above is an example of this, as the dog which had the puppies was clearly "owned," as she spent most of her time in the neighbour's yard.

34. Saunders, T., & Storr, D. (2002). Op. cit.

35. The Nassau Guardian (1970). Tropic topics. 18 April, p. 4.

36. Lockwood, R. & Ascione, F. R. (eds.) (1998). *Cruelty to animals and interpersonal violence*. Purdue University Press.

37. The Tribune (1999). Animal abuse an early warning sign, Humane Society officer says. June 16, p. 5.

38. The Punch (2003). Nicki Kelly Between the lines. 8 May, p. 16.

39. Health Information Unit. (2001). *Bahamas youth health survey*. Ministry of Health, Nassau. Unpublished. Due to the high level of non-response to some questions, the percentages of the entire sample (1,007 replies) are given.

40. Jorgensen, S. & L. Maloney. (1999). Animal abuse and the victims of domestic violence. In *Child abuse, domestic violence, and animal abuse*. Ascione, R. & Arkow, P. (eds.). Purdue University Press. 143–158.

41. For example: The Tribune (2002). Doctor's advice after 'alarming' child abuse and neglect figures. 31 July, p. 2, and The Nassau Guardian (2002). Woman charged with cruelty to children. 30 August, p. 7A.

42. For example, The Nassau Guardian (1991). Animal cruelty in Pinewood. 21 June, p. 8A.

43. The Tribune (2002). Pets in dander from poisoners. 12 May, p. 3; BBC News (2001). Op. cit.

44. Hubrecht, R. (1995). The welfare of dogs in human care. In: *The domestic dogs: Its evolution, behaviour and interactions with people*. Ed. Serpell, J.: 179–198. Cambridge University Press.

45. Hubrecht, R. (1995). Op. cit.

46. The Nassau Guardian (2003). G.B. Humane society highlights incidents of animal abuse. 2 May, p. A5.

Chapter 15: Health Issues Related to Dogs

1. For example: The Tribune (1999). Stray dogs: A complicated problem. 25 February, p. 10.

2. Beck, A. (2002). Personal communication.

3. See also The Tribune (2000). Pet of the week. 8 July, p. 10, which concerns a dog found in a school's grounds.

4. See p. 128 above.

5. According to WF's daughter.

6. Beck A. (1973). *The ecology of stray dogs: A study of free-ranging urban animals.* Purdue University Press, reprint.

7. We have already noted that this may primarily be due to heartworm.

8. Ownby, D. (2002). *Journal of the American Medical Association* 288: p. 963. Reported in New Scientist (2002), Pets train your kid's immune system. 175 (2359). P. 24.

9. From our census of the veterinary clinics (see Table 4.2).

10. This approach was later justified when roaming dogs in a poor area of Nassau killed a resident. See Chapter 16.

11. This is not a clear economic distinction, but residents with health insurance can be expected to visit private clinics.

12. This compares with 53% of households who fed dogs they do not own and 77% of households who reported roaming dogs in their neighbourhood, Table 8.2.

13. This apparent confusion reflects the perception of ownership noted earlier.

14. Casley, D. J., & Kumar, K. (1992). The collection, analysis, and use of monitoring evaluation data. Johns Hopkins University Press, Baltimore. Third edition.

15. The Freeport News (2002). Students treated for scabies. 27 September. Pp. 1, 3.

16. Households which claim to own a dog or that have dogs in the yard which they do not claim to own.

17. Data supplied by the Ministry of Health & Environment (2001).

18. Data supplied by the Ministry of Health & Environment (2001).

19. Animal Sheltering (2001). BARK may lead to fewer bites. March–April, pp. 3–7.

20. Weiss, H. B., Friedman, D. I., & Coben, J. H. (1998). Incidence of dogs bite injuries treated in emergency departments. *Journal of the American Medical Association* 279(1): 51–53.

21. Weiss et al. Op. cit.

22. For example, North Americans own about 1.3 dogs; Ralston Purina (2000). The state of the American pet—A study among pet owners. Ralston Purina.

23. The Nassau Guardian (2002). Rodent problem can only be curbed through "education." http://nas.bits.baseview.com/nas_templates/print/280183751955206.nas.

24. Powell, T. (2001). Personal communication. Environmental, Sanitation and Consumer Protection Division, Department of Environment Health Service, Nassau.

25. Mather, J. & Fielding, W. J. (2001). The threat posed to personal health by dogs in New Providence. *Bahamas Journal of Science* 8(2): 39–45.

26. Jones, K. (2001). Personal communication. Deputy Registrar, Office of Vital Statistics, Department of Health, Florida.

27. Davis, A. C. (1999 & 2001). Personal communications. Animal Care & Regulation Division, Broward County, Florida.

Chapter 16: Dog Bites

This chapter uses dog bite data classified as E 9060. For example, Injury Missouri Information for Community Assessment documentation and definitions. http://www.health.state.mo.us/Injury/allinjurydef-doc.html.

1. The Tribune (2001). Minister: we're tackling dog issue but public must help. 19 September, p. 6.

2. Data supplied by Medical Records Department, Princess Margaret Hospital, Nassau.

3. Patients not requiring to be admitted.

4. According to Edwards, J. (2002). Personal communication. Medical Records Department, Princess Margaret Hospital, Nassau.

5. Gershman, K. A., Sacks, J. J., & Wright, J. C. (1994). Which dogs bite? A case-control of risk factors. *Pediatrics* 93: 913–917.

6. Rottweilers are also one of the most popular breeds imported into The Bahamas (Table 10.2).

7. Sacks, J. J., Sinclair, L., Gilchrist, J. Golab, G. C., & Lockwood, R. (2000). Breeds of dogs involved in fatal human attacks in the United States between 1979 and 1998. *JAMA* 217(6): 836–840.

8. Gershman, K. A., Sacks, J. J., Wright, J. C. (1994). Op. cit.

9. The Nassau Guardian (2001). Strange attack not the work of potcakes. 11 September, pp. 1A, 3A. There are unconfirmed reports that an owned pit bull and rottweiler were actually responsible for the woman's death, although potcakes were also close by.

10. The Tribune (1991). Attack dogs must be handled with care. 29 November, pp. 1, 15; The Tribune (1993). Pit Bull mauls child to death. 15 May, pp. 1, 8; The Tribune (2001). Woman savaged by pack of dogs. 10 September, pp. 1, 11.

11. For example: The Nassau Guardian (1993). Stricter control for dog owners. 19 May, p. 1.

12. The Tribune (1991). Man dies after being mauled by guards dogs 21 November, p. 1 The story of the death of Rudolph Penn is included in a general crime roundup. Interestingly, his death seems not to have provoked any discussion on the use of guard dogs to protect property.

13. "Potcakes are not generally considered dangerous dogs. In fact, they have a mild temperament and are generally considered loveable and loyal." The Tribune (2000). Packs of wild dogs pose major problem. 20 November, p. 3.

14. Turnquest, S. (2001). Personal communication, Bahamas Humane Society.

15. The Nassau Guardian (1987).Pit bull menace. 1 July, p. 4A. Problems with breed specific legislation are discussed by Armstrong, M. C., Tomasello, S. & Hunter, C. (2001). From pets to companion animals. In: *The state of the animals 2001*. (ed. Salem, D. J., & Rowan, A. N. Humane Society Press, Washington. 71–85.

16. The Tribune (1994). Letter to editor: Law banning pit bulls should exclude guard dog industry. 20 April, p. 4.

17. The Tribune (1993). Letter to the editor: Laws to make dog owners responsible needed here. 20 May, p. 4.

18. The report in The Nassau Guardian (1991), Dog bitten man dies at hospital, 22 November p. 3A, states that a pit bull and a potcake were involved. Our interviews with those involved with the incident revealed that both dogs were pit bulls.

19. The Nassau Guardian (2001). Strange attack not the work of potcakes. 11 September, pp. 1A, 3A.

20. The Tribune (2003). Letter to editor. 1 July, p. 4; The Nassau Guardian (1987). Vicious pit bulls upset family. 29 April, pp. 1A, 3A. Although pit bulls are not a recognized breed by the Bahamas Kennel Club, they are perceived to be a breed by some people. See, for example, The Nassau Guardian (2003). Pets for sale advertisement, "Purebreed pitbull puppies . . ." 27 June, p. B4. A pit bull breeding with another type of dog would then be considered by some to be a cross-breed.

21. We know of two "breed" pit bulls which were abandoned by their owner near the airport in September 2002. The owner had let them loose, as he could not "cope" with them anymore.

22. See, for example, The Tribune (2001). Minister: we're tackling dog issue but public must help. 19 September, p. 6; The Nassau Guardian (1993). Public urged to become responsible animal owners. 5 October, pp. 3A, 4A; The Tribune (1993). Pit bulls must be banned from Bahamas. 21 May, p. 4; The Nassau Guardian (1998). Stray dogs seen as "a people's problem." 8 May, pp. 11A, 15A.

23. The Tribune (2003). Letter to the editor. 1 July, p. 4.

24. Leny, J., and Remfry, J. (2000). Dog population management. In: Macpherson, C. N. L., Meslin, F. X., and Wandeler, A. I. (eds.), *Dogs, zoonoses and public health.* CABI Publishing, UK, 299–331.

25. The Punch (2002). Letter to the editor: Ban pit-bulls before dogs kill a tourist! 15 October, p. 30.

26. In January 2003, a tourist was badly bitten by roaming pit bulls in Harbour Island. The Tribune (2003). Tourist in dog attack horror. 29 January, pp. 1, 11.

Chapter 17: What Future for the Potcake?

1. Anon (undated). What is a potcake? http://www.biminilove.org/potcake.htlm.

2. The Tribune (1924). Recently organised Bahamas Humane Society. 10 December, p. 6.

3. The Tribune (2001). "CCU need help to tackle dog nuisance." 17 October, p. 5.

4. JM knows of a well-meaning person who neutered the dogs of willing owners in a small community. While she maintained this service, there were almost no roaming dogs in the village. When she discontinued this service, within a few years the situation had reverted to what it was before she first visited the village.

5. JM knows of a group that had neutered roaming dogs which were later, unwittingly, caught by the Animal Control Unit and killed by euthanasia.

6. The Tribune (2002). Letter to the editor: Success of spray [*sic*] programme. 21 November, p. 4.

7. Leny, J., and Remfry, J. (2000). Dog population management. In: Macpherson, C. N. L., Meslin, F. X. and Wandeler, A. I. (eds.), *Dogs, zoonoses and public health.* CABI Publishing, UK, 299–331.

8. Hinsey, A. (1974). Presenting animals in the primary school. Unpublished project, Bahamas Teaching College (now The College of The Bahamas), Nassau.

9. The Punch (2003). Animal owners urged to be more responsible. 27 March, p. 41.

10. The Tribune (2003). Putting the bite on Grants and Bain Town dog problem. 2 July, p. 2.

11. Eighty-eight percent of the population claimed to be an active member of a church group in our 1998 perception study.

12. Due to the constraints of the school timetable, inclusion of any new subject must result in the exclusion of another topic that is also regarded as essential for the child to learn. Thus, the accommodation of pet care in a curriculum is not a trivial exercise.

13. This was confirmed by an enquiry at one of the larger bookshops in Nassau, which revealed that it had no books at all on pet care.

14. The Nassau Guardian (2003). The Mini page. Dogs! Dogs! Dogs! 7 February. Supplement.

15. The Nassau Guardian (2001). Editorial: New group to address stray dogs problem. 30 October, p. 8A.

16. For example, The Nassau Guardian (2002). Letter to the editor: Bahamians should be proud. 6 March, p. 6A.

17. The Tribune (2002). Letter to editor: Success of spray [sic] programme. 21 November, p. 4.

18. Anon (undated). Legislation dog owners should know. Department of Agriculture information sheet

19. Manning, A. M., and Rowan, A. N. (1992). Companion animals demographics and sterilization status: Results from a survey in four Massachusetts towns. *Anthrozoös* 5(3), 192–201.

20. Mather, J., and Fielding W. J. (1999). A report on the ARK spay/neuter programme in New Providence with suggestions for Government action. Submitted to Ministry of Agriculture and Fisheries, Nassau.

21. This also includes relatives of deceased owners. This matter was highlighted in a newspaper report. The Guardian (2003). Girls rescue toddler from vicious dog attack. 20 January. P. 1.

22. The Guardian (2003). Girls rescue toddler from vicious dog attack. 20 January. P. 1.

Appendix 1: Questions Used in the Pet Attachment Study

1. Templer D. I., Salter C. A., Dickey S., Baldwin R. & Veleber D. M. (1981). The construction of a pet attitude scale. *The Psychological Record* 31, 343–348.

Appendix 2: Notes on the Derivation of the Balance Sheet

1. From our studies; see Chapter 10.

2. Unpublished calculations by WF.

3. From our perception study; see Chapter 10.

4. The Tribune (2000). Pets in danger from poisoners. 12 May, p. 4.

5. Anon (undated). Report for the months of January–December 1999.

6. From our studies on garbage and handouts; see Chapter 8.

Index

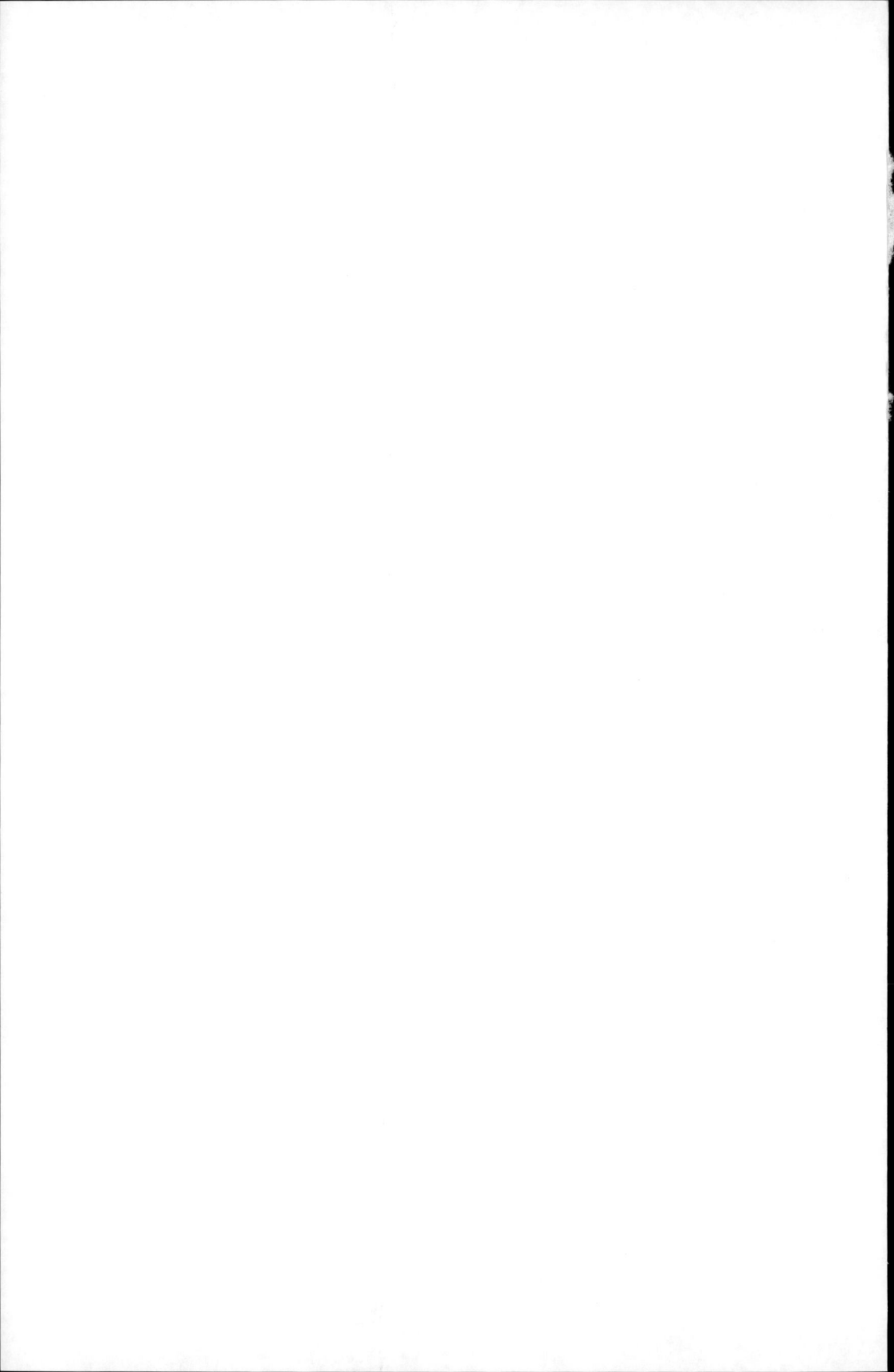